"Meredith O'Brien writes deftly and gracefully about the shock of becoming an unreliable narrator as she navigates both disbelieving doctors and the challenges of her own changing brain in the process of searching for answers to the concerning symptoms she experiences. A journalist by training and a writer by nature, she fearlessly investigates, contemplates, and confronts her diagnosis of multiple sclerosis as she learns to adapt to her body's new way of being in the world. Her frank look at what this process is like for both herself and her family will be heartening to anyone who has lived with the uncertainty of chronic illness."

— *New York Times* bestselling writer **Andrea J. Buchanan**, author of *The Beginning of Everything*

"In *Uncomfortably Numb*, Meredith O'Brien writes unflinchingly about her life before and after her MS diagnosis. Detailing her treatment, her struggles to be taken seriously by doctors, and the effects of it all on her family, career and sense of self, she writes in a clear-eyed and courageous voice, bringing the reader along with her as she navigates this profound, life-altering experience."

— **Sarai Walker**, author of *Dietland*

"*Uncomfortably Numb* tells a sadly all-too-common story: of a woman whose symptoms were initially dismissed by doctors before a life-changing diagnosis. Frank and relatable, it will speak to anyone who knows the uncertainty that chronic illness brings and the resiliency it demands."

— **Maya Dusenbery**, author of *Doing Harm: The Truth About How Bad Medicine and Lazy Science Leave Women Dismissed, Misdiagnosed, and Sick* and writer/editor Feministing.com

"A candid, in-depth look at one woman's journey with MS and how it touches those around her. A great read for anyone struggling with chronic illness from diagnosis, through acceptance and into thriving in the new normal."

— **Lori Espino**, president of Greater New England chapter of the National Multiple Sclerosis Society

"Poignant and thoroughly readable, *Uncomfortably Numb* is a deeply personal look at how the diagnosis of a debilitating illness such as MS profoundly affects patients and their families. It is also the story of a strong woman who is learning to adapt and is determined to persevere."

— **Cathy Chester**, speaker, writer of MS blog An Empowered Spirit

"*Uncomfortably Numb* is a rare window into everyday life with multiple sclerosis, and how chronic illness can turn one's very identity inside out. The illness is unpredictable: an initial diagnosis takes years to materialize, symptoms may or may not signal the progression of the disease, and treatments are imperfect. With candor, O'Brien bares her most vulnerable moments as she learns the new rules of working, parenting, and living in the present when the future is uncertain."

— **Jessica Fechtor**, author of the bestselling memoir *Stir: My Broken Brain and the Meals That Brought Me Home*

"A modern telling of the newly diagnosed story from a no-nonsense journalist, a gifted writer, a pragmatic New Englander. While uniquely her own—by definition—there will be few who have or know chronic illness who will not glimpse well-told aspects of their own experience in this memoir. *Uncomfortably Numb* is heart-breaking, it's harrowing, and it's heroic."

— **Trevis Gleason**, author of *Chef Interrupted: Discovering Life's Second Course in Ireland with Multiple Sclerosis*

"A memoir penned with such truth you won't know if you should keep reading or pause to shed a tear. O'Brien showcases the individual effects of the debilitating reality for those facing multiple sclerosis. Not only does the author tackle the painful veracity of the disease, but provides reminders of how critical the healthcare system is to those in need."

— **Savannah Hendricks**, author of *Grounded in January*

"O'Brien writes with the measured curiosity of a journalist and yet with a raw vulnerability, giving an honest, unflinching look at navigating life with chronic illness. *Uncomfortably Numb* is a triumph that will take readers on an emotional journey and leave them with hope."

— **Elissa Grossell Dickey**, author of *The Speed of Light*, blogger for National MS Society

"Uncomfortably Numb pulls readers into the reality of an unexpected and life-altering diagnosis of multiple sclerosis, with forthright clarity, detail, heart, and insight. O'Brien's memoir is not only a gift to adults dealing with MS, but also for people grappling with any other sudden onset diseases and similarly 'invisible' conditions—and for the people who love them. An engaging, thought-provoking, informative story, and a narrator you'll want to know and follow."

— **Lisa Romeo**, author of *Starting With Goodbye*

"A riveting memoir...O'Brien's honesty, humility and humor will have you flying through the pages, rooting for her every step of the way."

— **Joan Dempsey**, author of *This Is How It Begins*

"O'Brien's tenacity shines through on every page. While managing the MS she continues to work, takes care of her...parents, and raise her children. The author refuses to give in to the many challenges that life throws her way. An inspiring read."

— **Diane Cook**, author of *So Many Angels: A Family Crisis and the Community That Got Us Through It*

"Meredith writes clearly and honestly about the painful stages of shock, recognition, and acceptance that you go through when you learn you have a chronic illness. Throughout, she never loses sight of what's really important in life—her family and her own identity as a writer."

— **Rose Pike**, executive vice president of editorial at Remedy Health Media

"Meredith O'Brien's journey is beautifully expressed in reality that only someone with MS understands—a must read for anyone with multiple sclerosis or connected to MS."

— **Caroline Craven**, writer, blogger and MS life coach at GirlwithMS.com

Uncomfortably

Numb

Uncomfortably

The life-altering

Numb

diagnosis of

a memoir

multiple sclerosis

MEREDITH O'BRIEN

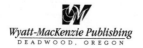
Wyatt-MacKenzie Publishing
DEADWOOD, OREGON

Uncomfortably Numb
A Memoir
The Life-Altering Diagnosis of Multiple Sclerosis
Meredith O'Brien

ISBN: 978-1-948018-70-8

Library of Congress Control Number: 2020931385

Neurons Font designed by @missjoyceli
Neurons cover image ©Burgstedt

Some of the material included in this book was previously published on the National Multiple Sclerosis Society's MS Connection blog. It is published here with the Society's permission.

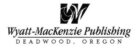

Wyatt-MacKenzie Publishing
DEADWOOD, OREGON

www.WyattMacKenzie.com

Requests for permission or further information should be addressed to:
Wyatt-MacKenzie Publishing
15115 Highway 36, Deadwood, Oregon 97430

Dedication

To my brother, who shares my twisted gallows humor

Table of Contents

BEFORE

AFTER

Preface

Everyone lives with a ticking clock. A finite future. Actually, it's more than finite. It's unplannable, sometimes unimaginable.

I used to like to think that with thoughtfulness, careful attention to one's choices, and proactivity, a person could create the blueprints for one's life and adhere to those plans. That's what I used to think. I saw it all quite clearly in my head: I would finish college, get married to my college sweetheart, get a job as a newspaper reporter, attend grad school, start a family. Everything went according to plan until my body stopped cooperating and sent my husband and me through infertility treatments. After years of uncertainty, I had twins who were born five-and-a-half weeks prematurely and who spent weeks in the neonatal intensive care unit. They were too fragile for me to leave in order to go back to work full-time, so I became a freelance writer and adjunct faculty member, teaching journalism at my alma mater. Three miscarriages in the span of eighteen months followed before I gave birth to our third child. At this point, I no longer believed in blueprints. Life, I concluded, was a combination of what happened to you and how you reacted to random events, to things you pursued, and to opportunities you were afforded.

Just when I dared to consider attempting to plan my future once more, fate had other ideas. In a matter of months in 2014, I unexpectedly had a job change, my sixty-five-year-old mother died of cancer, my father fell seriously ill, and I received the life-altering diagnosis of multiple sclerosis, an incurable neurological disease of the brain and spinal cord. MS is a wild card. No one can predict which course a patient's MS will take. At least not yet. I had been in the process of writing the book about a middle school jazz band in mourning when MS symptoms settled over my world like an omnipresent fog.

Will I ever be able to finish this book? I asked myself. *Will I ever be able to teach again? Will anyone want to hire me? Will my family, including my three teenage children, forever see me as someone who's sick? Will this insert an unwanted caretaker/ill-spouse dynamic into my marriage?*

A year after the diagnosis, I decided to write about having one's life upended. This book chronicles my transformation from being a relatively healthy woman to someone whose life was transformed by illness. *Uncomfortably Numb: A Memoir* allows readers to accompany me on this journey, from the moment I realized I had numbness in my left leg, to the years-long diagnostic process that, at times, made me feel as though I was insane, as at least one neurologist suggested my symptoms were a manifestation of my long-standing anxiety issues.

One of the biggest questions with which I wrestled after learning I had MS was the question of whether I'd be able to finish writing the book about the school jazz band—about which people in my town were routinely asking me as it was about the local middle school band members grieving the loss of a peer—before I got really sick ... if I got really sick. Would MS prevent me from completing it? Would my course of the disease hinder my verbal abilities, my reasoning, my thinking? I didn't have the answers to these questions and had no blueprints on which I could rely.

Interspersed with medical reports, physician's notes and information from the National Multiple Sclerosis Society, *Uncomfortably Numb* introduces readers to the world of confusing acronyms, foreign-sounded medical jargon, and the realm of demyelination with which I was contending. At times, the medical records confirm my suspicions (when, for example, I didn't think a doctor believed what I was saying). In other cases, the records and MS information explain things I didn't fully understand at the time (like the fact that hanging out in hot and humid weather would, at least temporarily, make me feel very ill). Text messages I exchanged with family and friends, as well as in-person interviews helped me fill in the blanks. My current neurologist—whose name, along with every other medical professional mentioned in the book, has been changed—also sat for an interview.

Four medical memoirs served as inspiration: Susannah Cahalan's *Brain on Fire: My Month of Madness*, about a twentysomething newspaper reporter's hard-to-diagnose brain infection; Jessica Fechtor's *Stir: My Broken Brain and the Meals that Brought Me Home*, about a PhD candidate's nearly fatal brain aneurysm and her long recovery; Suzanne Strempek Shea's *Songs from a Lead-Lined Room: Notes—High and Low—from My Journey through Breast Cancer and Radiation*, about a former journalist-turned-novelist's cancer treatment; and Andrea J. Buchanan's *The Beginning of Everything: The Year I Lost My Mind and Found Myself*, about a writer who had a cerebrospinal fluid leak that incapacitated her for many months until it was finally repaired. All four of these writers provided readers ringside seats to how their medical conditions altered their lives, their views of themselves, their bodies, their relationships.

In the process of writing this, I read books by other MS patients. Ann Romney's *In This Together: My Story*, Kristie Salerno Kent's *Dreams: My Journey with Multiple Sclerosis*, and Marlo Donato Parmelee's *Awkward Bitch: My Life with MS* gave me much to think about, including how the disease affects each patient differently and interrupts the patient's life with terrifying swiftness.

By the time readers get to the final page, my hope is that they will not only understand the impact of chronic and incurable diseases, but will appreciate the importance of having something that pulls you forward, motivates you to get out of bed in the morning, regardless of how you're feeling.

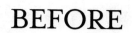

BEFORE

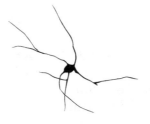

CHAPTER ONE
Someone Else's Leg

There's something weird going on with my leg.

I realize I'm not supposed to be focusing on myself, but this leg is really distracting me. I'm supposed to be devoting my attention to this middle school jazz band director sitting across from me in a practically empty T.G.I. Friday's on a summer afternoon in the Solomon Pond Mall in Marlborough, Mass. I'm supposed to be actively listening. Several weeks earlier, I started a new writing project where I would shadow Jamie Clark—an exuberant, public school music director with an affinity for bad jokes and bear-hugs, and who looked unnervingly like a shopping mall Santa—and his middle school jazz band during the 2012-2013 school year in the wake of the untimely death of one of the students, a twelve-year-old trumpet player named Eric Green. My elder son Jonah, age thirteen, is among the grieving members of that jazz band I will follow.

This mid-day interview in a chain restaurant is part of an on-going, years-long process of getting to know Jamie, the man who I only knew from afar as I watched him emcee the middle school concerts for Jonah's sixth and seventh grade years. He always struck me as a larger-than-life character out of a movie, as wildly outgoing, in stark contrast to me, a somewhat introverted journalist and writer who gets uncomfortable in crowds of people. Right now, he is telling me about how he doesn't hide his emotions from his students, how he will weep in front of them, that he's a sunny optimist at heart. I'm trying to hide my astonishment. I've taught students at the collegiate level for some time and, while I may joke around, I do not veer away from the professional demeanor I present in the classroom. I would *never* cry in front of them.

We could not be more different.

"You can choose your attitude," the prematurely gray-haired and bearded forty-four-year-old band director tells me before diving with gusto into his ample lunch, a double cheeseburger with extra cheese, which takes up all available real estate on his plate. He says he wants to role model this positive attitude, for his students, who are in mourning and who miss their pal Eric who unexpectedly died in his sleep in January 2012. During the upcoming school year, he says, he's going to need to figure out a way to help his young musicians channel their raw emotions through their instruments. I try to imagine Jonah channeling his feelings through his drumsticks, but I cannot.

A friendly-looking man—except when his students forget their sheet music or their pencils, in which case, his warm blue eyes turn icy—Jamie pulls two necklaces out from beneath the crew neck of his light blue "Life is Good" T-shirt which says, "Big Kid" and depicts a stick figure of a man jumping into royal blue water. He's showing me the charms on the necklaces, a Celtic Triskele—a symbol of the "triple Goddess" of the maiden, mother, and crone, which some people interpret the symbol as meaning life, death, and rebirth—and a Celtic circular symbol which he says represent eternity and re-birth. "Whatever you put out there comes back to you. ... These are physical reminders of what's important," he says, messily finishing off his burger.

I am taking notes old school, by hand, in one of my many steno notebooks with the light green pages and am trying to maintain a professional mien, not reacting positively or negatively to what he's saying. I'm supposed to be Switzerland. Neutral. That's what I was taught in journalism school. I'm there to gathering information and to try to understand what and why things occur in order to paint a complete, contextual picture for my readers. However, as I am sipping my second Diet Coke (which had been preceded by two cups of coffee that morning), I notice something is off with my left leg. Beneath the booth, I brush the calf of my right leg across my left shin, both of which are bare because I'm wearing capri pants. It's August in New England, thus it's hot and humid outside, but, because the restaurant's air conditioning is turned way up, I am comfortable. But something doesn't feel right on that leg and I can't stop thinking about it. I brush my left calf across my right shin to compare the sensations. The right leg is positively brimming with feeling.

Yeah, not right, I observe silently as I continue scribbling down what the high-spirited, verbose band director is telling me. I say nothing about my left leg.

After an over two-hour interview, I exit the mall and pass through a wall of heat threaded with significant humidity as I walk to my car. Now that I'm alone, I can fully focus on how odd the skin on my left shin feels, of how my feet feel in the brown leather slide sandals with the cork wedges, of how the hem of the linen capri pants feels as though it's rubbing evenly across my right shin and calf, but not so with my left. Inside my beat-up, black SUV, the heat is suffocating. I turn on the air conditioning as high as it will go and lower all the windows to let the heat escape so I can breathe.

As the air turns from hot to cold, I close my eyes and focus on my legs.

Does it feel different on my left? Does it really? Is this like it was before, just something strange that will just go away?

⤺

When I was a twenty-four-year-old newspaper reporter working in western Massachusetts, there was a one-week period where the surface of my left arm felt numb. Not completely numb. Not pins and needles either. More like a diminished sensation. It was subtle, but atypical for me. I made a mental note of it but didn't freak out. Attempting to be tough and single-minded, I continued with my work, making phone calls from my gray, metal desk in the Westfield bureau of *The Union-News*, trying to reach officials in the tiny town of Southwick, Mass., the community that juts out from the straight southern edge of Bay State that eventually morphs into the arm-like shape of Cape Cod.

A few days after the arm numbness appeared, half of my face felt numb too. That same diminished sensation. Like Novocain wearing off after a dental procedure. I could still move my features and feel my lips if I touched my fingers to them. The fact that numbness was taking over more territory like a conquering army gave me pause and made me wonder what was happening. It was like a minor mystery that needed to be solved rather than something potentially worrisome happening to my body. I figured a doctor would be able to provide some answers.

I conferred with my husband Scott who was working at an engineering firm on the opposite side of the state. He seemed more concerned than I was. Alarmed, would be a good way to describe him. "Call a doctor," he said with a sense of urgency.

By the time I was examined by a doctor a few days later, the odd numbness had abated but he ran tests anyway. He found nothing awry and issued a clean bill of health. I wrote the whole incident off as no big deal and moved on.

$\backsim$

Fast-forward to 1997 when I was twenty-eight. Scott and I were living in a Marlborough apartment now, having recently moved back to our home state of Massachusetts from the

Washington, D.C. area. We had moved down to Maryland so I could attend graduate school at The American University, where I earned a master's degree in political science and worked as an investigative journalist while Scott worked as a transportation engineer. Life in D.C. was filled with our exciting work (him on transportation projects, me reporting on presidential candidates), following politics like it was a spectator sport, going to Happy Hours with work friends at local watering holes like the Brickskeller and the Mad Hatter, and taking weekend trips around the D.C.-Maryland-Virginia area to Colonial Williamsburg, Annapolis, Baltimore, and Virginia Beach.

When we talked seriously about starting a family, we decided we'd move back to Massachusetts where both of our families resided. The plans we were making, our expectations of how our lives were going to unfold, were shattered when I could not get pregnant. More than a year of humiliating tests to figure out why this wasn't happening, followed by increasingly invasive infertility treatments involving regimens of intermuscular shots at various tender spots in my body yielded nothing but bitter heartache, bloating, and empty arms. Because of how involved these treatments were—on some weeks I had daily bloodwork and frequent ultrasounds—when we moved to the Boston area, I decided to seek part-time work as a journalism professor and freelance writer so I'd have scheduling flexibility. Scott found a full-time job in a Boston suburb.

When I wasn't teaching, planning lessons, or writing, I was left alone in our apartment to stew in my thoughts, which were becoming increasingly despairing and frustrated. Joining an online bulletin board for women experiencing infertility issues was the only thing that provided me with a tenuous tether to sanity. These virtual strangers seemed to me to be the only ones who understood the emotional impact of infertility and the sudden realization that having a family would not be a given. To the rest of the world—where it seemed as though the vast majority of people could seemingly get pregnant at will—all was fine with me, with Scott and me. We didn't let on the anguish behind our poker faces, the feelings of failure and fear. Other than the online strangers, only a handful of people in my inner circle knew what was really happening and how Scott had learned to wield a hypodermic needle like a pro.

It was in the middle of these treatments when the right half of my face froze. Looking in the mirror was like gazing into an abstract painting. I would smile but only the muscles on the left side of my face would respond. The right side remained impassive, ignoring the signals my brain sent to my nerves. I attempted to raise my eyebrows, but I only looked half-surprised. Chewing with half a mouth became an ordeal as I tried to avoid chomping on my own tongue (the right half of which I couldn't really feel) or having crumbs accidentally spray out past my lips. So on top of the hell of pumping hormone shots into my body, of my hopes for a baby being dashed month after month after month, half of my face had become unresponsive.

I tried to keep it together, to not crumble, to remain calm.

Again, I went to see a general practitioner who quickly diagnosed me with Bell's Palsy, a temporary malady which strikes an estimated 40,000 Americans yearly. The National Institute of Neurological Disorders and Stroke describes it as "facial paralysis resulting from damage or trauma to the facial nerves." A cursory internet search I did after being told I had Bell's Palsy yielded images of asymmetric faces looking as if half the flesh had slipped off skulls, melted in the sun like wax off a candle. Not. Comforting.

It's temporary, just temporary, I repeatedly told myself like a meditation mantra, hoping that the students to whom I was teaching journalism wouldn't notice either my facial asymmetry or my slightly slurred speech. While I had had no trauma to my face or head—none of which I was aware—I accepted the diagnosis and prayed for whatever was wrong to right itself back again.

My lowest moment amid this unexpected life curve, was when I still had partial facial numbness and learned that another cycle of fertility treatment had failed. No pregnancy. No baby. No answers. No reaction in the right half of my face. Scott came home from work to find me sitting on the floor next to our sofa in our darkened basement apartment crying, an empty martini glass on the banged-up coffee table he and a friend had made when we were in college.

Scott put his briefcase on the kitchen table and squatted down to embrace me, unsure as to what he could say to offer comfort.

"I just want this to work," I sobbed. It was a bursting of the dam, a reaction to the helplessness induced by a body that wouldn't cooperate, by the mystery of why this was happening, by my inability to fix it. I didn't like this. I was embarrassed by my watery sobs. I was a hard-ass reporter. A planner. I liked to know what was going to happen and when. I liked to prepare and be prepared. The combination of these events stripped away my sense of control, even if it was really the illusion of control.

True to everything I read online, feeling gradually returned to my face over a period of weeks, as did my natural, nasally speech. The only thing that was truly "off" about my face was my slightly crooked nose, but it's been crooked for as long as I could remember. That, I could live with, the sense of a lack of bodily control the infertility and the Bell's Palsy created within me was another matter entirely.

⌣

Days after my interview with Jamie Clark, when I first noticed numbness on my left leg, I run a disposable razor blade down my left shin. Water from the showerhead above sends the tiny, shorn hairs down the drain beneath my feet. As I watch the hair disappear down the drain, I realize it feels as though I'm shaving someone else's leg. It's not that I can't feel the pressure of the blade on my skin. I can, but just barely. If I don't look down, I can't discern if the blade is touching me. The best description I come up with is this: imagine shaving when you're wearing a pair of tights. You'd still feel the blade travel down your leg, but not clearly. Alarmingly, over the course of a few days, the diminished sensation in my flesh heads downward, toward the earth, affecting the top and outer edge of my left foot. It heads skyward too, moving all the way up to my outer thigh. Always a good rule of thumb: if numbness is spreading, consult a doctor.

Feeling very déjà vu-ish about this traveling numbness business, I call my general care practitioner, assuming that by the time I'm examined, everything will be normal, just like it was nearly two decades ago.

On August 16, 2012, the day of the appointment, I am forty-three years old and am sitting, fully dressed, atop a thin sheet of white paper on an examining table in a nondescript suburban health center. It's the same medical center I visited when I had a similar complaint about numbness in my arm and face when I was a twentysomething newlywed. The paper crinkles as I squirm and begin to sweat, even though there's air conditioning and I'm wearing light clothing. My genial physician, Dr. Thatcher* (names of all medical professionals have been changed)—a long-haired middle-aged woman who seems as though, in different circumstances, she could very well become a friend—starts asking questions, like whether I'd sustained any injuries recently. All I'm looking for are clues as to what she thinks is happening to me as the numbness has not gone away.

I already have my suspicions. I'm a reporter at heart. A researcher. It is rare for me to walk into a situation blind. This approach can have both benefits and drawbacks. Drawbacks include me reading a long list of potential causes of my symptoms and then catastrophizing, wondering what my life would be like if I have X, Y, or Z, which leads me to silently panic, which then transforms my stomach into fleshy, painful knots. The benefits of my journalistic approach include me having a battery of questions at the ready.

Prior to walking into my primary care doctor's office, I searched the internet for likely reasons for leg numbness, an option that wasn't available when I had arm and face numbness in the early 1990s. By relying only on legitimate medical sites—like the Mayo Clinic and the National Institutes of Health (NIH) —I narrow down possibilities: a herniated disc/pinched nerve, Lyme disease (I see no visible bite marks, but ticks are so small that I may have missed a bite), and multiple sclerosis. I am leaning toward herniated disc because I've had mild back issues. I'm not too worried though.

Dr. Thatcher says she's going to order a panel of blood tests, looking for Lyme disease and issues with my thyroid. She also orders an MRI, something I've never had.

Wait, an MRI? I think. This gets my attention as a shot of adrenalin pulses through my veins.

I arch my left eyebrow. "An MRI? Looking for ... what?"

"Well," she stammers, avoids making eye contact.

"A pinched nerve?" I pause, trying to camouflage my nervousness. When she doesn't reply right away, I add, "MS?"

Upon hearing this, she looks directly at me. "Yes. We'll wait and see what the blood tests and MRI say."

An MRI that looks for multiple sclerosis is done of the brain and the spinal cord. She wants to look at my brain?!

Trying to counteract the anxiety that is now surging, I try to self-soothe, tell myself that it's likely Lyme disease. That's the only thing that could make sense.

After allowing lab techs to siphon off several vials of my blood, I resist the urge to Google multiple sclerosis on my smartphone as soon as I get back to the car. Even though I know it is one of the possible reasons for my symptoms, I don't want to delve any further. I worry about the powers of my imagination. If I start Googling things and possibilities I can't unread, it'll be like a starting gun has been triggered for my imagination to race down all sorts of potential avenues which will likely send me into a panic.

I'm not going to jump to that, I tell myself. *I cannot jump to that.*

⮑

The blood tests are negative for Lyme disease, an ailment that's quickly spreading throughout the Northeast. Scott and I are usually vigilant about putting a tick-repelling ointment on our dog Max on a monthly basis. If we miss an application by, say, a week, it's very likely that the short-legged, shaggy tan and black Havanese-Wheaten Terrier mix will bring several creeping insects into our house. We have already removed a great many ticks that nestled between his thick tufts of hair over the years, a feat that require multiple people to hold Max down and for someone with a steady hand to yank the blood-sucker out of his flesh with tweezers. My younger son, Casey, who used to love playing in the woods that surround our yard, once had a tick lodged in the back of his head where his curly, sandy-colored hairline ended, and his bare neck began. That tick dug in so deeply that his pediatrician had to numb the area before extracting the remnants of the pest with a surgical instrument. Even though I didn't think I had experienced a tick bite, Lyme disease had seemed like a realistic possibility. But now that this is officially off the list of culprits, I am averse to thinking about the unsavory option that's left.

I book my initial MRI for August 22 at eight-thirty a.m., noting to myself that the numbness has continued to slowly creep across my flesh like wild ivy, wrapping itself around my entire left leg and left side of my abdomen. As the numbness advances, I am starting to quietly obsess about what the MRI will find, fretting about the possibilities while I lie in bed at night pretending to sleep.

For most people, having an MRI—an acronym for Magnetic Resonance Imaging, a scan involving gigantic magnets that move around but never touch the patient—is just another scan. One friend told me he took a nap during his only MRI but he's much more laidback than I am. Couple my claustrophobia with immobilizing my head by putting a Hannibal Lecter-type of a contraption over my face, two inches away from my eyes in order to achieve an accurate brain scan, and that's a recipe for a panic attack, something I'm apt to have on occasion, particularly in crowds or confined spaces. A therapist has helped me with the panic attacks and anxiety over the past few years and I feel pretty good about the progress I've made and the tools I've learned to employ in stressful situations. But with something like this, involving physical restraints and small spaces, I fear my brain chemicals will overwhelm me, so I take a mild sedative beforehand. By the time I arrive at the MRI facility, I have already taken the chill pill and am doing my best to pretend I'm unfazed by the whole thing.

As I undress in the patient changing room, I am blissfully ignorant that I'll soon have a face contraption placed on me. I am likewise unaware that, in order to scan my brain—I think they are going to scan my neck—I need to lie motionless, in a narrow tube that is laughably called an "open" MRI. It's slightly wider than a birth canal. Had I researched brain MRIs (which I did not, likely an unconscious move of self-preservation), it would have been very hard for me to remain calm and fight the potent urge I have to snake my way out of the apparatus as soon as the scanning begins.

A kind technician, Bob, ushers me into the wide room with the gigantic machine in the center. It's a beast of a behemoth with a hole in the middle.

Where my head is going to be, I think.

The people who will be doing the scan are behind a wall that's half-glass. Their voices are only audible to me if they flip on a microphone. As I climb onto the narrow scanning bed that will be elevated and then deliver me into the maw of the magnetic contraption, I wish I was behind the glass with the technicians, chatting it up, maybe enjoying a turkey sub and some barbecue chips with Bob instead of lying on my back, being transported, head-first, inside an unknown future. This is *before* Bob puts cushioning next to my ears (to prevent me from moving) on top of the earbuds which are piping news reports (my choice from their listening options) that I will not be able to hear once the machine starts going. Bob firmly clicks the hard, plastic face cage into place. In some places, this thing is actually called a *cage.* Others refer to it as a mask. Cage seems more accurate because, once it is placed over my face—leaving a narrow, rectangular opening located over my eyes—I feel trapped.

If I wanted to, can I get out? I wonder, unable to move my head or look down to see how narrow this cage thing is at my neck, whether there's any wiggle room if I decide to bolt.

Bob—of whom I'm now wildly envious because he gets to move about freely and has a full range of vision—places this small, gray, rubber bulb into my sweaty hands. It is attached to a cord. If I squeeze it, Bob tells me, he'll get me out of the machine immediately. My personal panic button. But I'm skeptical. Surely my squeezing of this bulb, which reminded me of the nasal aspirator I used on my babies to clear their noses when they were sick, would not result in an *immediate* release from my confinement. There would be a delay, I am convinced. These negative thoughts pig-pile on top of my mounting angst about being trapped inside a machine that will scan my brain, the place where I store all my secrets, my fears, my desires, my aspirations, things I don't share with anybody.

They can't read what I'm thinking or what areas of the brain I'm using, can they?

My breath is getting shallower as I recognize the folly of my paranoia that the lab techs can read my mind.

If they could read my mind via an MRI, surely I would've read about that in the New York Times, *I think. This isn't a sci-fi movie or TV show where the government uses technology to peer into one's brain contents. This is real life. Stop being an idiot!*

My chest feels heavy. There's nothing directly pressing on it, but it feels as though I'm experiencing pressure, particularly as Bob sends the scanning bed upon which I'm now resting, inside the tunnel. I hear soft, mechanical whirring as the machine swallows me up. I close my eyes because I honestly do not want to see how close the walls are to my body. I do not want to see the lights. I do not want to see, via a mirror clipped onto my face cage, the reflection of Bob and his cohorts, free and unencumbered behind that glass wall.

I just want out.

Eyes clamped so tightly closed I'm likely forging new lines in my face, I listen hard for the news reports coming through the earbuds. I can hear the confident, full voice of the male anchor. Bob informs me via a speaker that the first scan will start in a few seconds. "It will last a couple of minutes," he says. "Please don't move."

Here's something they don't tell you before you are loaded into an MRI: the thing makes the most otherworldly racket you've ever heard. The thunderous nature of the magnets—which are spinning around you, combing through your tissues, bones, and organs—makes your body shake, like you're inside a giant cocktail shaker.

I sure could use a cocktail right about now, I think.

The noises astound me and completely drown out the newscast that sounds as if it's being beamed to me from inside a tin can someplace on the other side of the planet. Each different scan, examining a different slice of my brain from a different angle, comes with its own, warped soundtrack. I try in vain to locate a melody or rhythm but can't. One scan emits a sound like the rapid-fire strumming of a single note on an electric guitar accompanied by one pump of an accordion. Another reminds me of the repeated sounds of a drumstick on a snare drum, which vibrates only on my right side. Then there's the scan that makes me think I'm in a nightmarish loop of computerized error messages being chimed over and over again. My favorite: the one that sounds like angry protesters have gathered around the outside of the machine and are pounding on it, trying like hell to get inside. I feel the machine shaking, hear the menacing thumps and really, really have the urge to flee. Plus, my face is starting to perspire but I cannot wipe the sweat because that damned cage is in the way and I've been asked to remain still. Although I can feel a cool waft of air traveling the length of my body, my face remains hot as I squeeze my eyes even tighter. I can still see the flash of lights through my closed eyelids.

I'm on that wacky Willy Wonka boat ride and I'm not getting a chocolate factory at the end.

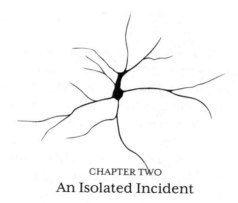

CHAPTER TWO
An Isolated Incident

I have a new job.

When I went in for the interview, I thought it was only for a position to teach a single writing class. It turned into a full-time offer. Sure, it's only a temporary full-time position—a two-year gig—but it's a temporary full-time teaching gig at a university located a short distance from my house. I'm told it has the potential of becoming permanent. It will be the best commute I've ever had and is way more convenient than those one-hour-forty-five-minute treks I took each way to and from another university to teach journalism classes part-time.

At this local university, I'll be teaching freshmen writing, an introductory journalism course, and will create an online and social media writing course, in addition to serving as a faculty adviser to the weekly student newspaper, where I'll attend Tuesday night meetings and help them edit the paper late into the evening on Thursdays. At the same time, on three mornings a week, I'll be observing seven a.m. jazz band rehearsals at the middle school in my town, Southborough, twenty-five miles west of Boston, as well as doing interviews for the book about the jazz band in mourning. All three of my three-season athlete children will be attending the middle school starting in September. I'll have two eighth graders and one sixth grader. Our lives will be riotously chaotic. And I am thrilled.

I sign the official job offer in August 2012. Since I hadn't been in a classroom for at least a year—I took a break from teaching to write a novel—I buy some new clothes, a new laptop bag, and an assortment of office supplies as I simultaneously pick up items from my children's long school supply lists. When I show up for faculty orientation at the suburban campus, I'm wearing my new red, sleeveless blouse—it is very hot outside, although I carry a very English professor-looking white lace sweater with me—along with a comfortable black skirt and shiny new Mary Jane-style pumps with little leather rosettes on the sides. In the conference room on the main floor of the student center, new faculty members —including the guy who will be my officemate—gather. I unpack my leather folder, my fresh notebook, and my excitement as I settle into a cushioned chair. After teaching on a part-time basis and being a freelance writer since my three children were born, it is a rush to have a full-time job like this one. We meet the university president, the dean of students, the university attorney, the head of HR. We talk benefits and syllabi, parking passes and university goals. Over lunch—where I eat only dry salad because, as someone with a dairy allergy, I can never be sure of the ingredients in the bread or the spreads on the sandwiches but usually don't ask people about the ingredients because I don't want to make things difficult or call attention to my allergy—I learn tidbits about my new colleagues including the fact that there's another baseball fan in the group, a history professor who's an Orioles fan, with whom I will exchange friendly smack talk when Baltimore plays my beloved Boston Red Sox. Upon the conclusion of the welcome sessions, several of us walk down to the campus police office together to get our university IDs—in mine I'm smiling broadly, and my face still bears remnants of a Cape Cod sunburn. We part ways with the new school year full of opportunity in front of us.

I climb into my SUV, blast the AC, and head home via back

roads. A minute or so into my drive, my cell phone rings. It's Dr. Thatcher's office. I'd called the office a few times since my MRI to see if they'd received the results, but they hadn't. My numbness, as of this point, has finally stopped encroaching on new areas of my body. The flush of excitement from orientation wanes the moment I see the medical center's name on my cell phone. I pull off the road and into the parking lot of a local country club so I can write down what the nurse tells me and not run off the road.

"Can you read the results for me?" I ask after I've put the car in park.

"Well ..." There is a long pause, the kind of pause a patient usually hears from a nurse who is reluctant to share information she's not sure she's authorized to share.

She tells me there is a large growth, "a mass," at the base of my brain on top of my spinal cord. This is not at all what I am expecting to hear. What I expect and want to hear is, "Everything's fine, but you have a small pinched nerve ..." The word "mass," in any medical context, is never good.

"Cancer?" I ask, my voice involuntarily squeaking.

"No ..." she says haltingly. She advises me to obtain copies of the MRI on a disc and consult with a neurologist. They think I might have multiple sclerosis.

The day that started with promise, a new job, a new school year, new clothes, new notebooks, new colleagues, ends in bleak fear in a country club parking lot.

～

I cannot stave off my curiosity. I've always been curious, wanting to know things, wanting to be the person who knows things, and wanting to be the one who tells others about the things I know. As a young girl, in addition to writing short stories in spiral notebooks I found around the house—detritus from my parents' truncated college days—I carried my mother's oversized gray tape recorder around, recording "news" segments, like interviews with my younger brother Sean who told scary stories about a kid he knew who once forgot to get off the school bus and who was taken back to the bus depot. I recorded myself reading front page stories from the local newspaper, for which I'd later become a news reporter. My neighbor Gina would come over and we'd pretend to be a TV news duo. We'd allow Sean to participate in the news show only in the capacity of a meteorologist named Walter Cronkite. My parents used to tease me about this penchant for gathering and distributing news, nicknaming me the Bad News Bear, that's when they weren't calling me Mere-Bear, a cutesy moniker I came to despise by the time I was a teenager.

After hearing news of the "mass," I pull out my laptop when I get home and search the internet for information about multiple sclerosis, knowing, full well, that by doing so, I cannot un-know whatever I may find. I will not be able to extract the fear that will be lodged in my gut once I look at some of the websites. I will not be able to stop envisioning what my future might look like if I have this disease. My vivid imagination will take this information to all sorts of places when I try to go to sleep at night. Nonetheless, I click on the first legit source that crops up, figuring the National Multiple Sclerosis Society should know its stuff.

"Multiple sclerosis (MS) is an unpredictable, often disabling disease of the central nervous system that disrupts the flow of information within the brain, and between the brain and body," the site says. I focus on the *often disabling* part. "The cause of MS is still unknown—scientists believe the disease is triggered by as-yet-unidentified environmental factors in a person who is genetically predisposed to respond. The progress, severity and specific symptoms of MS in any one person cannot be predicted. Most people with MS are diagnosed between the ages of 20 and 50, with at least two to three times more women than men being diagnosed with the disease." The site does an excellent job of breaking down the nuts and bolts of the disease, using scientific language buffeted by basic explanations. "Multiple sclerosis (MS) involves an immune-mediated process in which an abnormal response of the body's immune system is directed against the central nervous system (CNS), which is made up of the brain, spinal cord and optic nerves." In essence, the site says, the protective nerve insulation (myelin) is destroyed, and that destruction interferes with the communication between the damaged nerves and the brain and spinal cord.

But what about that disabling business? Do I really want to know how bad it can get? I ask myself, knowing it won't be hard for me to envision worst-case situations. *Yes,* I decide, *I want to know.*

Most common symptoms, according to the National Multiple Sclerosis Society, include: fatigue, walking difficulties, numbness or tingling, spasticity, weakness, vision problems, dizziness and vertigo, bladder problems, sexual problems, bowel problems, pain, cognitive changes, emotional changes, and depression. Less common symptoms: speech problems, swallowing problems, tremors, seizures, breathing problems, itching, headache, and hearing loss. There are photos of smiling people in wheelchairs, photos of people using arm braces to get around.

I am a writer and a teacher who reads all the time. I could lose cognitive function? My vision? My hearing? My ability to walk about in front of the class? Around the campus? What would this mean for my life? For my husband who'd have to deal with something for which he didn't bargain? What about my kids?

I stop reading. In fact, I close my laptop. I don't want to know any more. I've read enough. And besides, no one has told me I actually have MS.

⌒

The neurologist with whom I get an appointment in Boston has asked that I get another MRI right away. This news is as welcome as a Tabasco enema. This MRI will be just like the first, with the odious face cage, then, while I am still lying on my back, a contrast dye will be injected into a vein in one of my arms. The contrast dye—a substance called Gadobutrol— enables physicians to see organs with more clarity, particularly if they are inflamed. In the case of MS, there may be inflammation in the areas of active nerve damage. Right after my brain is scanned, I will be slid out of the tunnel on the narrow bed, admonished not to move as the cage is removed from my face and moved down several inches to cover my cervical region so images can be made of my neck and upper spine both with and without the contrast solution flowing through my veins. This will give the doctors a better look at what is going on and whether that "mass" they found is what is called an active MS lesion.

Unfortunately, Bob isn't going to be the one helping me, soothingly speaking to me through the intercom while I try to envision myself on the other side of that glass wall, eating chips and talking about last night's Red Sox game. Bob's MRI facility does not have any openings so I have to book an MRI at another location and bring the scans from the new facility with me to my September 25 neurological appointment, a little less than a month into my first semester in my new job. In another unfortunate coincidence, the second MRI is scheduled for August 31, the day after a retreat for English department faculty who teach writing, where we will discuss techniques, syllabi, and lesson plans. As I meet my new colleagues for the first time, I have to stuff my worries that I may be diagnosed with a disease with no cure into a box, lock it, then sit on top of it to make sure none of the fears escape and sully the positive impression I'm laboring to make. I can't really assess how things are going. I tend to have a lousy poker face, but I'm trying to project enthusiasm about this job opportunity, not raw fear that my life is about to potentially explode. Things are going well for me professionally right now, with the book project and this new job. I don't want anything to get mucked up, so I pretend I'm not fretting about the next day's MRI. However, the juxtaposition of the two—a new beginning and a dire, uncertain health prognosis—is weighing on me.

My second MRI is a mid-morning affair. I am on edge and take a sedative. After the previous day of play-acting as though everything is fantastic, acting like the head of the English department made a brilliant choice in hiring me, my emotions are precariously close to the surface, a tsunami lurking beneath the phony, toothy smile. I miss Bob. Bob is a nice dude, a compassionate one. Not so the tech I have for this hour-and-a-half appointment. Ninety minutes. On that damned table. Without moving. Half of it with an IV in my arm sending contrast dye through my veins while a face cage keeps my head stationary. The head with the mystery "mass" inside it. The mass I've been trying not to think about. Every minute. Of every day.

Maybe this woman Verna is having a tough morning. Maybe she received some ominous health news herself recently that she hasn't revealed to anyone either and she's trying to keep her cool while she's at work. I try to imagine what's going on in her life that could be making her so disagreeable. I don't know what her deal is but she is holding in her hands the doctor's order so she knows what mine is. Despite that, she gives me curt directions and handles me the way a teenage clerk handles produce at the grocery store checkout line. She abruptly clicks the face cage into place after making sure the earbuds, piping jazz music into my ears (I figured I'd try to see if music would help) are out of the way. She doesn't have any extraneous discussion me. She unceremoniously hits the button that sends me away, into the magnetic tunnel, without so much as a word.

The cacophonous symphony of the MRI overloads my senses as well as the jazz I am straining to hear. I slam my eyes shut tightly again and try to envision myself somewhere else. But it can't be a vague somewhere. It's got to be specific. A beach on Cape Cod—in Wellfleet to be specific—pops into my head. It's LeCount Hollow, down a short dirt path from the Wilson Avenue cottage my parents used to rent for a large chunk of my youth and young adulthood. It's on the Atlantic Ocean. There's a strong saltwater breeze. There are tiny fuchsia rose buds on the bushes clinging to the weathered gray, split-rail fence in the front yard. I imagine the grit of the sand that, despite my mother's frequent sweeping, is never entirely absent from the cottage floor. The mosquitos—which always find their way through the worn window screens and eventually chew up my exposed skin they seem to love—are buzzing near my ears. I imagine it all. I am there, out of this cage, where I do not have a mass in my brain. There are no pounding sounds of the machine which is shaking as it tries to read the innards of my body and tell me what they're saying. There's just the sound of the surf and those mosquitos.

With abruptness, Verna pushes the button that delivers me out of the tunnel. She grabs my right arm, swabs it with an alcohol wipe and inserts the IV before loading it with the contrast dye. I flinch because the needle stings. I more than flinch. I adjust my leg as I flinch.

"What are you doing?!" Verna yells. I can't see her face because the cage is blocking my view. "You can't move! You have to stay in EXACTLY the same spot, or we can't compare these scans to the other ones otherwise we're wasting our time!"

That is all I need. The seal on the dam is ripped off, broken. The flood is unleashed. I am crying. I hate crying in public, in front of anybody. Hate. It. I avoid it at all costs, preferring to let loose, all blubbering in private. And this one, man, it is one ugly cry, the kind where your nose runs and turns a flaming blotchy red, where your eyes get puffy. To add to the humiliation, I have to let my nose run and allow the tears to roll down the sides of my head, where they moisten my hair and mouth. I cannot hide my face because I cannot move. My fear is naked. I am exposed.

Verna sees me and something in her softens. "What, are you scared honey?"

"This test is to find out if I have MS."

"Oh," she says, "okay honey." She stops chastising me. She pats my hand with three, rapid touches, pushes the button that sends me back into the tunnel, then retreats behind the glass wall where no one is crying.

I am inside the tube trying desperately not to move, lest I further "ruin" the MRI scans as tears flow from my eyes unbidden.

⌇

School starts for my three middle schoolers and me. As they meet their new teachers, I acquaint myself with the college campus, find best spots to eat (food that I can eat without being poisoned because of my dairy allergy), to get coffee (the bigger the better), and to read my dead-tree newspapers comfortably in a spot of sun. I set up my shared office with my new colleague, place a Boston Red Sox decal on the window in front of my desk, and situate photos of Scott and kids on the windowsill, marking the territory as my own. I meet the student newspaper staffers and start attending editorial meetings and editing sessions. (Mega-sized portions of coffee are required to make it through the newspaper editing, I quickly learn.) I create writing prompts and assignments, attempting to persuade my freshmen writing students to open themselves up and to tackle subjects about which they really care, to tap into something authentic. I want them to prove to themselves that they have something to say and, deep down, they know how to say it. I'm building their self-confidence while mine is packed away on ice awaiting the appointment with the neurologist.

I am not breathing a word about what may or may not be going inside my head, about the worry that has lodged itself deep in my bowels, taken up residence, suppressed my appetite, and caused chronic stomach discomfort. I don't tell anyone about the "mass" other than Scott and my college roommate and closest friend Gayle, who lives outside of Boston. Not my parents (not yet anyway), not my kids, not fellow parents I see on the sidelines of soccer and hockey games, not the middle school band director Jamie of whom I am asking all manner of private and probing questions about his life, his philosophies, his objectives. The irony of this is not lost on me. On top of this, the Red Sox are on their way to last place in the American League East which, to me, is a major bummer. To distract myself, I focus on the teaching, on my book research, and on my kids, a sixth grader, Casey, and my eighth grade, boy-girl twins, Jonah and Abbey.

I wait for weeks before I can meet with the neurologist and learn his assessment of the second MRI and what he thinks is happening to me. The appointment is at six-fifteen in the evening at the end of the day when I teach three classes, two of them back-to-back. I am cranky, tired, and scared. I picked this neurologist because of his hospital affiliation, not because I know anything about him other than the fact that he is a board-certified neurologist. My general practitioner, Dr. Thatcher, didn't have any recommendations so I searched for physicians at trusted Boston hospitals.

I ask the six-feet tall, booming-voiced Scott to accompany me into the exam, which, in hindsight, is a mistake. His presence seems to undermine my credibility with this doctor, who, I'm guessing is in his late thirties or early forties. Dr. Sabine winds up talking to Scott a lot more than to me after I share with him that I just started a new job, have three children, and tend to be an anxious person in general. After taking a detailed medical history, we move onto the physical exam to evaluate the numbness I tell him I have. Dr. Sabine takes out a short pin and touches its sharp end to my left leg and foot. He asks me to tell him how much sensation I experience, from nothing to full sensation, on a scale of one to one hundred, like whether I have fifty percent sensation or ninety percent or one hundred percent. This kind of scale doesn't work well with me. I'm not a numbers person. Having to assign a numerical value to the level of numbness throws me, therefore my answers are uncertain. I want to be correct, but want time to think about the level of sensitivity. He wants an immediate response. Instead, I'd rather indicate to the doctor the areas where I am experiencing diminished sensitivity, which has spread no further upward than my abdomen and stretched down to the front of my left ankle. We are trying to communicate in different languages, on different planes. I don't think my wordy explanations are resonating with him. Dr. Sabine examines my eyes and their movement. He watches me walk, tests my reflexes, has me touch my index fingers to my nose in rapid succession.

His determination: I have one lesion on my brain stem. (So, we've moved from calling it a "mass" to a "lesion.") He says he has no idea how old the lesion is, but the MRI did not show it to be active. In fact, the MRI didn't show any additional lesions. "Multiple sclerosis is multiple lesions," Dr. Sabine says. He continues: "MS doesn't usually present like this. You have an unusual pattern of numbness that doesn't really conform with multiple sclerosis." He looks to Scott and nods affirmatively as if this all makes sense. In a pleasant, friendly voice, Dr. Sabine tells me to keep up with the yoga I am doing, urges me to de-stress myself, and to see him in January. As I walk out of there, I know I should feel relieved, but I don't. I get the distinct feeling that he doesn't believe that I'm experiencing numbness. Shame fills me as my face flushes.

Years later, I read Dr. Sabine's medical notes from our initial meeting and they confirm what I felt in the room. Despite the fact that the MRI found a "single lesion in the c-spine," described as a "hyperintense lesion in the central/anterior spinal cord at the C2 level, just below the cervicomedullary junction, approximately 10mm in length," and that a physical exam found "decreased sensation to pin," Dr. Sabine wrote, "She does have a history of anxiety with panic attacks, and has been under significant stress recently; a psychosomatic manifestation is certainly a strong possibility ... The lesion noted on the brain/cervical spine imaging is unlikely to be related to her numbness."

There it is. In writing. I was being completely forthright, admitting anxiety—which we are frequently told is nothing be ashamed of—and my admission was used against me. I was dismissed as just another nervous chick. Nothing to see here. Despite that mass thing. Anxiety doesn't yield brain masses, last time I checked.

According to the National Multiple Sclerosis Society, what I'm experiencing is something called Clinically Isolated Syndrome, where there's one lesion: "Clinically isolated syndrome (CIS) is one of the disease's courses. CIS refers to a first episode of neurologic symptoms that lasts at least 24 hours and is caused by inflammation or demyelination (loss of the myelin that covers the nerve cells) in the central nervous system (CNS)." If a patient with one brain lesion found on an MRI that is "similar to those seen in MS," the society says, "the person has a 60 to 80 percent chance of a second neurologic event and diagnosis of MS within several years." Dr. Sabine didn't tell me any of this, never uttered the phrase "clinically isolated syndrome." He suggested I return in several months and we'd see where we were.

In early January 2013, with one semester of full-time teaching under my belt, I see Dr. Sabine again. I have new areas of numbness including on the back of my left hand, across my fingers, and on my wrist, while the leg numbness has started to dissipate. Dr. Sabine seems unconcerned by what I'm saying and tells me I should see him in a year and adds, "if anything new crops up."

I am confused: *Do I see him in a year only if I have symptoms in a year? But isn't this hand and wrist numbness new? Why does he keep asking me about anxiety?*

A note written by Dr. Sabine to Dr. Thatcher after the second appointment, reveals what I sense from his tone: "Since her last visit, she has had a mild subjective increase in numbness in the left dorsal hand, without any other symptoms. Her repeat MRI done recently is unchanged, with no new lesions. ... While I strongly suspect that her numbness is psychosomatic in origin, a multiplex small-fiber neuropathy would be another possibility."

He thinks it's all in my head.

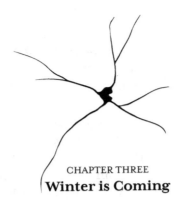

CHAPTER THREE

Winter is Coming

It's an unseasonably warm autumn day, as I'm driving home from the university on a late Thursday afternoon in October 2013, a little more than a year after I experienced that weirdness with my left leg. Since the embarrassment I felt upon leaving Dr. Sabine's office and feeling as though he didn't believe what I had been experiencing, the numbness I felt has largely gone away. That makes it easier to try and forget about the whole matter, the stress-inducing MRIs, the loss of sensation on my body, and the "lesion" in my brain. I am focusing, instead, on my second year of teaching, on writing the book for which I've recently concluded reporting, and on my two high school freshmen and my seventh grader.

On this Thursday afternoon, I've got a tiny sliver of time between the end of my last class and when I need to be back on campus to help student journalists edit their weekly newspaper. I usually wind up staying on campus until midnight or later, on Thursday evenings. Today, I'm racing home so I can whip up a quick dinner for the kids before I leave the house again. Maybe I'll pry some tidbits of information out of them, like how the cross country or soccer practices were this afternoon for Jonah and Abbey, or how seventh grade lunch fared for Casey. My boys constantly accuse me of interrogating them because, after their content-free answers to my questions about their days (Questions: "Did anything interesting or funny happen today? What was the best or worst part of your day?"

Answers: "Nope." "Dunno."), I follow-up with specific questions, drilling down until they cough up something of substance.

"Stop being an investigative reporter," Casey is fond of saying, as though this is going to stop me from asking questions.

"If you just give me something, talk about something specific, I won't have to keep asking you more and more questions," I say.

As stubborn as the boys can be, I can match them with my own muleishness.

All the parenting literature I've read up until now, urges parents to maintain open lines of communication with our teens, suggesting that on a regular basis we should learn about their friends and about how their classes are going. The literature doesn't tell us how difficult and infuriating that task can be. It doesn't tell us HOW to extract that information from recalcitrant kids who just want to flee the moment a parent starts asking questions. (It must be noted here, that Abbey does not flee and, in fact, offers up information about her day without being interrogated. I frequently point this out to her brothers, suggesting they adopt her technique, but they blow it off and accuse Scott and me of treating her like the MFC, the Most Favored Child.)

Anticipating typically vague answers from Jonah and Casey, I'm trying to use the time in the short car ride home to come up with some new lines of inquiry and develop a conversational road map when my cell phone rings. It's my father. *He never calls at this time of day*, I think. As I hit "speaker" on the iPhone, I'm ill-prepared for what's to follow.

"Mere, I've got some bad news. Your mother is in the hospital."

My sixty-four-year-old mother started hemorrhaging the previous night from her groin. The bleeding was so profuse that my father called an ambulance. This woman—who was thrown into menopause in her early fifties by chemotherapy for stage three breast cancer—had been experiencing menstrual-period-like bleeding for months. But she kept news about this bleeding to herself. She didn't seek medical attention until the blood was coursing out of her. Now, my father tells me the ER doctors who initially saw her are saying they think she has cervical cancer. They say they could see the tumor with their naked eyes.

I look out the passenger side window, stunned, and notice I am next to the local country club, the same location I'd been passing when I received the call about the "mass" in my brain a year ago. My first reaction, I'm embarrassed to admit, is fury. Absolute fury. Back in 2000, my mother Judy—a five-foot-ten, formidable, striking woman with dark hair and penetrating brown eyes, who runs two wine and liquor stores in western Massachusetts—waited a year before seeking a medical opinion about a large lump in her breast. At age forty-nine, she'd never had a mammogram and hadn't seen a doctor in years when she discovered the lump. But Mom was frightened and made excuses to herself about what the lump could possibly be, knowing, deep down, that something was wrong. When she finally saw someone after she turned fifty, she received the news she'd been afraid she'd hear: Breast cancer. With my twin toddlers in tow, I booked her to see a breast cancer specialist in Boston. Abbey, Jonah and I accompanied her to appointments. My father and brother Sean, who was in law school, waited together in the hospital waiting areas during her two breast cancer surgeries, listened as her surgeon told us her cancer had spread to her lymph nodes. Mom endured cycles of radiation and multiple rounds of chemotherapy to beat back the disease.

I would call her daily from my Boston area home every night to boost her spirits, keeping from her news of two of the three miscarriages I endured during her grueling treatment so as not to add to her angst. I became pregnant with

Casey during the end of her cancer treatment. When I finally told her I was pregnant, she held onto the promise of that pregnancy for dear life. She wanted desperately to meet this child, to live for this child, to hold him in her arms. And she did. Despite her tardiness in consulting physicians about that lump, she went into remission and was eventually declared cancer-free. Mom not only lived long enough to meet Casey—proudly walking a survivor's lap at a Relay for Life event while pushing him in his stroller, she also welcomed my brother Sean's three sons into the world, the last of whom was born in 2009. She, and we, were lucky. Her prognosis looked dire back in 2000. But she'd come out the other side.

And here we are, back in the same damn place. Mom had known something was wrong with her for some time but kept quiet.

"Why the hell did she wait?" I rage at my father, whose own voice is quavering. It is not one of my proudest moments. "Why didn't she see someone?! This is so stupid! I can't believe it!"

"I don't know Mere. You know your mother."

I call Scott and rage some more. "What was *wrong* with her? Why *did* she delay getting treatment? If they could *see* the fucking tumor, if it was bleeding to the point where parts of the tumor were sloughing off, it's got to be very advanced!"

I once again call the Boston hospital on Mom's behalf to book an appointment for her. In the meantime, a cursory internet search based on the information my father shared made me doubt whether she would be lucky the second time around. Before her appointment in Boston and against Sean and my vehement objections, Mom decides to have surgery to remove what we learn is not cervical cancer but is a grapefruit-sized tumor in her uterus. The procedure is done at a hospital closer to her home in the western part of the state—as opposed to in Boston, near where Sean and I live. Sean and I want her to see doctors who have a lot of expertise in this area, but Mom wants to proceed with getting that thing removed from her body immediately, and to do so locally.

The gruff surgeon, still in her scrubs after the procedure, tells my dad, my brother and me that Mom's tumor perforated her uterus and extended into her body cavity. It was a uterine sarcoma, an aggressive cancer. She estimates that Mom has about six months to live. Dad's face turns a deep red as he orders us, as well as the doctor, not to share the six-month prognosis with Mom, saying he thinks she'll give up on treatment if she hears this prognosis. I argue the benefits and morality of fully informing her of what we know, saying I'd want to know if it was me, although I'm not very aggressive with my assertions. In the end, I cave and defer to the parental authority.

There is no way, I tell myself, *that she doesn't know the severity of what's happening.*

With this news, I find it really difficult to push myself through my fury which casts a shadow over everything, over my teaching at the university, over the writing of the jazz band book now that my year of observation is over and I'm still digesting what I witnessed, over watching my children flourish. While I am featured at an Authors & Artists event at the university to discuss my new novel shortly after her procedure, my mother's cancer is there, lurking behind my false smile. The fact that the protagonist's mother in my novel—written well before this cancer diagnosis—died, weighs on me, almost to the point where I can't breathe. The potentially fatal news about Mom is omnipresent in my mind when I'm standing on the sunny-yet-damp sidelines of Abbey's JV soccer game at the high school, even when she does a forward-flip inbounds pass that entertains the crowd, as I fight back tears that threatening to burst forth seemingly out of nowhere. When I'm reviewing my notes for my book about a concert at which the middle school students performed in December 2012, listening to recordings of their performances, Mom's cancer pops into my thoughts when I hear the students play a delicate ballad. Tears. As I draw my red, puffy winter coat closer around me inside the rink where Casey is playing hockey on a Sunday afternoon, I use my iPhone to determine if I can arrange for a grocery delivery service to bring supplies to my parents' house, something my newly-retired father tells me they don't want or need.

Although my rational side knows it's a waste of energy, I become consumed with rage that Mom delayed obtaining help—suicide via procrastination, that the surgery didn't take place at a Boston hospital, that I felt like I was being robbed of the possibility that my mother and I could ever repair the cavernous breach in our relationship, cross over that craggy gap that kept us apart emotionally for years.

〜

She is taller than me. She is a woman in a largely male-dominated profession and is feared by many for her toughness and sharp words, while I, someone who is always smiling and trying to appease people, am feared by none. She overcame a childhood marked by harsh corporal punishment, while I was spanked one time. She is invested in style and fashion, while she often calls me a "ragamuffin" who was always in need of a mani-pedi. She has the olive skin inherited from her Spanish mother and she tends to tan deeply, while I have bright white English/Irish skin from my dad's side and tend to burn and peel after being in the sun too long. She adores shopping for clothes and buying things for the house, while I adore watching Red Sox and UMass basketball games, as well as buying books. She never doubts herself or apologizes to anyone, while I am overloaded with doubt and apologize for things that aren't even my fault. She eschews books and news articles, while I live for them. She has an exquisite palate for wine and finer foods—she appears on a weekly local radio station segment as the Wine Mother—while I regularly bomb her tests when she asks me what I smell and what I taste in a glass of wine; I serve my kids marinara sauce that I got from a jar.

Mom and I have never connected. We are too different. Our differences have always felt like a failure on my part, the reason why we never seem to click, like there was something wrong with me, something I could never fix. I'd be lying if I said I wasn't jealous of the fact that my younger brother Sean is *her* child, the one who is the tallest in the family, the strongest, the one who shares her olive skin tone, the one who is feared by some because of his size. Sean is exquisitely fashionable and into the finer things in life, has been so since he was a young boy and requested Izod shirts and Ocean Pacific gear, while asking that lobster to be served at his eighth birthday party. Like Mom, Sean never shows doubt and, during the year between graduating from college and going to law school, worked with her at one of the stores she managed, becoming her promising apprentice whose palate and fine sense of taste ran alongside Mom's.

"You're your father's daughter," she often says to me. It isn't meant as a compliment. It's filled with disappointment, edged with anger and resentment, with dismissiveness, with a lack of respect for my beta-ness compared to her alpha personality. She usually says that after she's just explained something annoying Dad has done.

I often wonder if, aside from the vast number of commonalities between Mom and Sean, one of reasons I'm the least favored child (LFC) in the family can be linked to two incidents. The first occurred when I was four and Sean was a newborn. Mom placed Sean's baby seat on the upper part of a shopping cart at a large department store. Being an energetic four-year-old, I hopped onto the opposite end of the cart, my feet landing on the bottom bar with as much force as a preschooler can muster. However, one of the cart's wheels was faulty, causing the cart to overturn, sending my newborn brother onto the linoleum floor where he fractured his skull. Doctors later told my parents they couldn't allow him to fall or hit his head for the first two years of his life, a Herculean request for an active boy who loved to run and climb. My mother, age twenty-four when she had Sean, had to hover over the boy, hold him, watch him, make sure nothing came in contact with his head. For two years. It's only natural that an extremely tight bond between the two of them was formed. Years later, when Sean began experiencing night terrors—he once told my parents during one of these nightmares that he could fly, which was a problem because we shared a room at the top of a steep set of stairs—she had him examined by doctors. I remember a lot of talk and worried looks exchanged over the dinner table about him getting a "brain scan" in order to assure her there was no lasting damage from that fall in the store. In family lore, this accident which fractured my brother's skull was my fault. It is an ongoing joke, referred to by my father as "the time Mere tried to kill Sean."

The skull fracture story dovetails nicely with the near-drowning story which took place years later. Sean and I—approximately seven and eleven years old respectively—were holding hands and jumping over the Atlantic Ocean waves as they washed up on a Cape Cod beach. It was coming on high tide, that period of time when what had been a sand bar an hour ago, suddenly develops depth. (I will note here that I have never been a strong swimmer and was once fished out of the town pool by a teenage lifeguard after I unwisely jumped off a diving board at a friend's urging when I was in junior high, years after the near-drowning story I'm about to tell. At age seven, Sean's swimming was sub-par as well.) While Mom and Dad were on the blanket on the sand—Dad reading a book, Mom tanning—Sean and I were playing in the water without incident and were not fighting, which, for my parents, must've been a nice break. Neither Sean nor I noticed that the tide rushing up onto the surf's edge was growing stronger as the water grew subtly deeper around us. Then a rogue wave hit our faces and wrenched our hands apart. Disoriented after my head slammed into the sand, I slowly rose and spit saltwater out of my mouth. I didn't see Sean in the roiling waters and panicked. I ran to get my parents. Dad sprang from the blanket and retrieved Sean from the water (he was coughing, but okay) while Mom shouted at me for abandoning my little brother. Thus, a second tale was added to the family canon, referred to as "the time Mere tried to drown Sean."

Now there were two strikes against me.

In spite of attempting to kill my mother's favorite child twice, Mom spent years of my young adult life pursuing a fruitless quest to remake me in her image. She tried to persuade me to dress "better" and to calm my "wild" hair. (I was a teen in the 1980s, when "wild" hair and gravity-defying hairspray application was in.) While my brother coveted brand name clothing, none of that mattered to me. I didn't have the same appreciation for being fashionable like Mom and Sean. As I became a young adult and her verbal persuasion didn't work, Mom used gifts as unsubtle nudges. And since I was short on cash in those days, her gifts kind of worked. After visiting Scott and me when we lived in Washington D.C. as I attended graduate school, for example, she noticed that my soft, flowy moss green winter coat was showing wear, particularly at the wrists. When she got home to Massachusetts, she mailed me a highly structured cobalt blue winter coat with shiny, faux brass buttons. Very much of a Naval Academy flavor. Totally not my style. I wore it anyway because Mom was being generous, because Mom was more fashionable than I was and perhaps knew better, plus, I wanted to please her. Over the years Mom would give me a Trollbead bracelet (to which I never added anything, although the one Mom had was full of those artsy beads), chunky necklaces, and sweaters with bold, primary-colored stripes from the same store at which she frequented, a brand she said I should buy because that's where she shopped. For years, I did indeed buy this brand of clothing because Mom told me I should. Few of the items she gave me were things I would have ever selected, however I never said anything about not liking them. I would never do so. I was a grateful gift recipient and, honestly, scared to say these weren't my style. It was easier to just say, "Thank you." So I did.

Always a youthful-looking and intensely beautiful woman, Mom coaxed me to start paying attention to my looks early on, particularly in the early 1990s when I was apt to wear flannel and baseball caps. On my thirtieth birthday, she gave me my first jar of Oil of Olay facial cream and told me it was time for me to start slathering it on my face and neck every night. A few months after Casey was born and Mom saw me eating some French fries off my twins' plates while we were in a food court at an outlet mall, she warned me that that was how her mother got fat, by eating off her kids' plates, so I stopped doing that. I also used the Oil of Olay she gave me, along with the perfume she got me, and donned the clothing and jewelry she bought me as well. I drank the wine she told me to drink (sometimes after she corrected me in front of wait staff in restaurants when I attempted to order a glass of "cruddy" wine). I was deeply appreciative of her gifts and thanked her for them. When I used the products and wore the clothes, I realized I would never be her, just like I would never have the kind of relationship she had with Sean. Wearing the blue coat with the brass buttons and spraying myself with Shalimar was never going to change that.

During Mom's first battle with cancer in 2000, Sean couldn't help her out much because he was busy in law school. Although I was teaching a journalism class and working from my home as a freelance writer while taking care of my twin toddlers, I tried to fill the most favored child role and endear myself to her. I called her every day and spoke with her for an hour as I made dinner, having already set the twins up in front of *Blue's Clues* with plastic bowls filled with Goldfish crackers to tide them over. I brought Abbey and Jonah, in their double-wide stroller, to her oncologists' appointments. I researched the disease, bought books on breast cancer, and made a list of questions to take to appointments, at which I took copious notes and recorded the discussions so Mom could listen to them afterward. I located breast cancer support groups in her area, but she didn't want to attend them because groups where you shared emotions with strangers wasn't her thing. I became Mom's go-to resource, her confidante, her ally, her shoulder to cry on. Dad, shell-shocked by her diagnosis, was often too emotionally precarious to be of much help. It felt as though it was all on me. During this period of time, I was the center of Mom's universe. I felt special and important in a way I'd never been with her before.

By the time she was told her cancer was in remission, Casey had been born and I was an exhausted mess. Those hour-long calls during my dinner prep hours became impossible, particularly when Casey wanted to be held as I cooked and would cause a loud ruckus that wasn't conducive to carrying on long telephone conversations while Mom drove home from work. I couldn't muster the energy to throw the three kids into the minivan and drive the hour-and-twenty minutes to her house as much as I did when I just had the twins. Casey didn't sleep through the night until he was three, so I was only quasi-lucid due to massive infusions of caffeine. I had also started teaching journalism again—after having taken a break from teaching when Casey was an infant—and was writing columns and freelancing. Scott started having a lot of night meetings he had to attend, meaning he wouldn't get home until late in the evening. I was speeding toward burn-out territory. Something had to give.

Mom, to put it bluntly, never forgave me for putting an end to our daily calls and for cutting back on the number of visits I made to her house on the weekends. A few weeks after I'd stopped calling every day—I was slowly scaling back the calls— she confronted me. "Why are you shutting me out?" she asked.

"I'm not. I just can't talk to you every night while I'm making dinner. Casey needs constant attention."

My attempts to normalize a once-a-week call and to have the kids see my parents once every month to six weeks, were met with disappointment and anger. All the good will I thought I'd established during Mom's cancer treatment evaporated, like a trail of smoke dissipating in the sky.

Our relationship became more tense a few years later when Scott and I broke from family tradition. Instead of spending a whole week of Scott's vacation time with my parents in a rented Cape Cod house as we'd done for our entire married lives, Scott and I decided to do something new in 2006: we scheduled a road trip to take the kids to New York City, Philadelphia, and Washington, D.C. We would see the Statue of Liberty, the Empire State Building, the American Girl Store, the U.S. Capitol, the Lincoln Memorial, the Spy Museum, and Sesame Place in Pennsylvania, where we'd visit with cousins who were my kids' ages. Upon learning that we planned to do something different for our summer vacation, Mom booked a rental in Wellfleet, invited my brother, his wife, and their new baby to spend the week with them, and told everybody else *not* to tell me about it. Even though we had a free weekend before our road trip when my family could have visited them at the Cape, when we could've gone to the beach with the family, the fact that we chose to use Scott's vacation time for anything other than going to Wellfleet was heresy. When I heard she was explicitly forbidding people from telling me she and Dad were going to the Cape, I directly asked her during one of our now-weekly phone calls, "So, when are you and Dad going to the Cape?"

"We're not," she said.

I had betrayed the family. And this was the price.

In a subsequent whispered phone call he made out of

Mom's earshot, Dad defied his wife and told me when they were actually going to Wellfleet. He gave me the address of the rental house and urged me to bring the kids there for a day anyway.

"I'm not going where I'm not wanted," I said tearfully. "And she doesn't want me there."

From this point on, my relationship with Mom was marked by mutual emotional distance and power struggles. She made many trips to visit my brother's family, who lived ten minutes away from my house, but wouldn't inform me that she was coming and would infrequently stop by. Many times, when I'd call my parents' house, I could hear her telling my father she didn't want to talk to me, to tell me she was asleep. Dad knew I heard her rejecting my call and apologized once he was out of the room.

Determined not to allow the deteriorating relations affect my mother's relationship with my three children, I still, on occasion, asked her to babysit so they could spend time together. This was probably a bad move. Mom and Dad were babysitting one summer evening while Scott and I attended a Red Sox game. Unbeknownst to us, Mom had arranged for my brother's family to come over and told Abbey and Jonah that they were to watch their cousins. Jonah, an ardent rule-follower at the time, wanted to make sure all of this was okay with Scott and me, so he told Mom he wanted to call us. Mom said there was no need to call us; she was his grandmother and we were all family, so there was no need for him to seek permission from anyone. But Jonah persisted; it was his thing, persisting. He grabbed a handset and ran to another room to inform us of Mom's plans and to ask if it was okay. Scott and I said it was fine and that he shouldn't worry. Once we stepped into our darkened kitchen that night, Mom asked what we thought about Jonah's call, voicing her incredulity that Jonah insisted he obtain our consent for family to visit, that he would question her authority in this way. Scott calmly said he was glad Jonah told us what was going on.

One thing about Mom. She doesn't like people to challenge her. Challenging her usually doesn't end well. So, when Scott said he was happy Jonah checked in, that was akin to throwing down a gauntlet. And my cowardly silence as I stood next to Scott—I too was glad Jonah wanted to keep us appraised of what was going on—made me complicit. We'd challenged the matriarch who didn't think she needed anyone's permission to have family visit her daughter's house.

In Mom's eyes, I had chosen sides, chosen my husband "over" her, "over" my family. She said I had "thrown my lot" with Scott's family instead of choosing my own. Mom and I endured several arduous phone calls with her insisting that I didn't trust her and with me saying this whole incident wasn't about trust, just about sharing information. From her perspective, I was her daughter, and she didn't need any stinkin' permission to do anything.

When I disagreed with that assessment, adding that I wanted Jonah to feel as though he could always run things by me, I crossed over that invisible line.

Peak iciness occurred at a springtime 2013 book event to promote my novel about a woman who overshared private details about her family on the internet and paid a personal price for it. My parents arrived late to the event. Then Mom heckled me. Maybe "heckled" is too strong of a word: After I'd read excerpts from the novel, a woman attending the event asked about similarities between the book's main character and me, a person who used to blog about my kids until they asked me to stop because they felt I was invading their privacy. At this point, Mom interjected and asked why I didn't exert the same restraint when I was in college and wrote columns for the student newspaper about my childhood and which mentioned her. Liquor salesmen who were trying to get Mom to stock their goods in the two stores she managed, would gleefully brandish fresh copies of the college newspaper in front of her any time her name came up in my columns. "You didn't ask *me* permission," Mom said.

I had no response to her question.

Despite all this meshugas, I always thought I had time, that we had time, to fix this somehow. That maybe, once the madness of raising active kids waned, once the kids were in college, I'd have free time I could spend time with her, and maybe we could fix what was broken, or at least make peace with our broken places.

A few months later, we learned about her sarcoma, the six-month prognosis, and none of these disputes mattered any more. The final winter of our relationship had arrived.

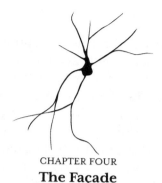

CHAPTER FOUR
The Façade

During November and December of 2013, Mom agrees to undergo harsh chemotherapy in Boston under the guidance of a uterine sarcoma specialist. The treatment robs her of her thick dark hair, strips her of her energy, and the healthy olive glow from her skin. It takes away the intimidation factor on which she used to bank because of her stature and her once-confident gait, particularly when she donned her towering heels. She agrees to receive painful injections of a medicine to bolster the growth of her bone marrow and to fight infection, injections which render her bedridden in the hours immediately afterward. She consents to staying overnight at my house on multiple weekends as I or my brother take her to treatments in Boston. She never once makes a crack about my less-than-stellar housekeeping, my choice of clothes, my hair, or the condition of my bath towels, things at which she absolutely would have taken aim if she was healthy.

The new year begins on an oppressive note because the winter weather has been brutal. Or perhaps it's just my mood that's making everything about 2014 seem brutal from the onset.

To the outside world, to my students, to my colleagues, everything seems fine. I seem like things are grand.

In January, I co-lead a faculty development session with a colleague—that Orioles fan I met at faculty orientation—about incorporating social media into the classroom. I talk about how, during my year-and-a-half at the university, I've guided students in using social media as a tool for creating and disseminating content, as well as for gathering information. During the presentation, I make jokes and smile so much that my dimples hurt. I think the presentation goes well, in spite of the fact that just prior to my session, I catch my heel on a step and fall down a set of stairs, feeling lucky that the cup of hot coffee I am carrying spills away from me and all over the stairwell wall. The bruises I get on my right arm and legs don't show up until later, well after the presentation has concluded.

In February, I head to New York City with Scott to see actor Bryan Cranston in his Tony-winning performance in "All the Way" on Broadway, where he plays President Lyndon Johnson during the fight for the passage of the Civil Rights Bill. As with many of the nighttime events Scott and I have attended over the past few months, I fall asleep halfway through "All the Way." Luckily, I'm able to hide my napping from Scott; he never notices me nod off. (I have very little memory of the play, something which greatly disappoints this history and politics buff.) I fell asleep during two other performances of other plays we saw in Boston during the past few months as I was inexplicably unable to keep my eyes open. I start to wonder if the stress of my mother's dire situation is sapping my energy and if that's why I am suddenly so very tired all the time. However, all seems great on my social media feed where I post a photo Scott took of me getting Cranston's autograph after the performance.

The smiles at the presentation, the joyous-looking social media posts are a façade.

Inside my body is where the truth lies. It's where my stomach is angrily churning on a regular basis. It's where I am starting to be aware that I'm grappling with a never-ending sense of fatigue weighing me down like a heavy blanket. It is getting harder and harder to get up early and work those late nights at the student newspaper. That numbness I experienced back in 2012 through early 2013—which Dr. Sabine suggested was psychosomatic—is starting to reemerge.

At the end of February, the Boston sarcoma specialist tells Mom, Dad, and me that a new uterine tumor has already replaced its predecessor that was surgically removed in October. This tumor is just as large as the last one. Fluid is quickly building up around it, causing my mother serious discomfort. The doctor does not recommend another surgery. Mom must know this cancer, unlike the previous one, cannot be stopped, but she doesn't acknowledge this to any of us. (Months later, when browsing through Mom's daybook I see this entry in the margins of the February pages: "The chemo is NOT WORKING!") Dad continues to keep secret from her the six-month prognosis.

The closest thing Mom and I have to an authentic conversation about this horrific development is one night on the telephone when she talks about the new tumor and allows herself a rare moment of vulnerability. As I listen to her, someone who looms larger-than-life in my world as an embodiment of female assertiveness and strength, discuss her fears—something I cannot recall ever hearing before—I am struck dumb. I have nothing brilliant or uplifting to offer this woman who had a very difficult childhood, who wears the sadness and disappointment of her youth around her shoulders like a shawl. I have no answers. I do not know what to say. I do not know how to comfort her. I cannot repair what has been broken. Our time has run out. I cannot turn myself into the daughter my mother wishes she had had, and I'm deeply devastated about that. Even bending the knee and playing the role of the good, placating daughter cannot offer Mom any solace now.

"I'm so sorry Mom," I say weakly, not wanting to cry, not on the phone with her. I will cry—sob actually—after I hang up the phone. But while she's on the line, I will just repeat my expressions of sorrow and offer her a listening ear. "I'm so sorry. I wish I could do something."

"I know," she says, her voice tight, knowing.

Despite the obviousness of her situation, Mom maintains a shroud of denial. The day before she is hospitalized for the final time, she asks me to take her shopping when my family is visiting her and my father at their house in western Massachusetts. She buys black Vera Wang leggings and Katy Perry brand false eyelashes to replace the natural ones which have fallen out. I don't question why she's making these purchases. I am just doing whatever she asks of me and trying to keep things light and easy. She never gets to use either the leggings or the eyelashes. When she's admitted to the hospital in Boston due to the excruciating pain she's experiencing as her abdomen fills with liquid generated by the tumor, we learn that her organs are shutting down and her kidneys are failing.

"We should just try to make her comfortable," her oncologist tells my dad, my brother, and me after two liters of liquid are extracted from her abdomen. Dad doesn't want Mom to know that the oncologist wants to simply give her comfort care. I disagree but don't have it in me to fight with him. The only point on which I do actively disagree is whether Mom's brother who lives in the Philadelphia area, should be contacted.

"Then she'd know it was the end," Dad says.

"Well ..." I reply, letting the sentence fall away. "He needs to come see her while there's still time." I directly act against his wishes and inform my uncle about what the oncologist has said and give him the hospital info.

On Mom's first day in the hospital, a two-person palliative care team enters her room with the intention of discussing pain management and end-of-life issues. Dad stands where Mom cannot see him so he can wave his arms and shake his head in a vain attempt to steer the team away from the subject of death, as if she doesn't see what's obvious to everyone else. The head of the team, a man in his thirties, seems perplexed by Dad's gesturing.

"What would you consider quality of life?" he asks her.

"I don't know," Mom responds, irritated. I can tell she doesn't like his tone which, to be honest, is a bit patronizing. Mom doesn't give quarter to those who patronize her.

"Well, what is important to you when it comes to your care?"

"I don't know," she repeats. She shoots him a dark "back the hell off" glare, the kind which, for decades cowed liquor and beer salesmen who entered her office. It is the glare that has the power to chill the blood in my veins when it is directed at me.

⤚

It's February 27. My mother is napping. A knit cap is covering her now-bald head. I quickly check email on my iPhone. Throughout her hospitalization, I've been able to teach all my classes at the university and still spend the late afternoons and evenings with Mom every day. I haven't told my English Department colleagues what's going on, except for my office-mate. In my inbox I see an email sent by the English Department chairwoman with the schedule for the fall of 2014. My name is not on it.

Over the past few weeks, I had been trying to schedule a time to meet with the outgoing department head to discuss the fall, given that my teaching contract expires at the end of this semester, but we haven't been able to find a time that works for both of us, especially since I have to leave right after classes to go to the hospital. I am thoroughly confused by the fall schedule. I send her a quick and, frankly, desperate email asking if this is an oversight because I really want to continue teaching at the university and really enjoy my work. My student reviews have been excellent and she herself has given me strong teaching evaluations after observing me in the classroom.

Via email she tells me "the department" has decided to go a different way. They want to hire people with terminal degrees, meaning the highest degree that can be achieved in any given field. In my case, that meant I had to possess either a PhD in English or an MFA in writing. I have a master's degree, but it's not terminal, and it's in political science.

By mid-May, I'm finished at the university and, like with my mother's illness, there's nothing I can do about it.

Later that night, I tell Abbey, Jonah, and Casey that Grandma is dying.

⤿

Mom always handled the money. I have memories from when I was a kid of watching Dad beg her for cash or for a blank check. She kept a tight rein over the finances.

"What do you need it for?" she'd ask him. "Do you *really* need it?"

He'd plead and, usually, she would relent. But she never shared information about their finances with him and, to this day, he knows precious little about them.

The subject of money leaps into Dad's mind as a group of family members linger around Mom's hospital bed in the shadowy light of a late winter afternoon.

"Judy, where's the checkbook?" he asks softly.

My mother—wearing her soft cap that covers her now bird-like head, her dark eyes sunken deeply into her skull encircled by grayish circles—has her eyes closed. She isn't sleeping. She's floating in between lucidity and madness, that's when she's not screaming out in pain. She is slowly losing her faculties as the drugs and the cancer have their way with her. One minute she's having a logical conversation about what the Russians are doing in Crimea, the next, she's getting out of bed and saying she has to climb the nonexistent stairs to the nonexistent closet. Or she is raising her fist as if to hit me in the face when I adjust her blankets, accusing me of colluding against her with the "people beneath the bed."

But she hears my father's question about the checkbook. You can tell because she responds, albeit slowly. She raises her clenched right hand, still bearing the perfect begonia red manicure she got for Valentine's Day. (Throughout her cancer treatment, she still got her regular manicures and pedicures.)

"I'll never tell you," Mom says in a menacing, low, grumble. She lowers her hand to the pink blanket and says no more about the subject.

꒰꒱

It's the afternoon of March 5. Mom is no longer responsive to questions, hasn't been for more than twenty-four hours now. She isn't eating. She isn't talking. Her breathing is a nightmarish rattling sound that comes from the back of her throat and emerges through her parched lips. Her brownie-colored eyes are unfocused and open to mere slits. Sean has slept in her hospital room for the past few nights, so she won't die alone. Dad has been sleeping on a sofa at my house and sobbing through his nights.

Mom's body has been retaining fluid at a rapid pace as the sinister tumor balloons her belly. For days, I've been massaging her hands, arms, legs, and feet with a pricey olive oil lotion that I picked up at a gift shop, trying to give her moments of physical comfort. I am no longer angry that she waited so long to tell someone about what was happening inside her. What I am now is bereft about this relationship unfulfilled. The only thing I can give her now is a tender touch of my hands.

I am alone with her in the room, sitting in a sliver of sunlight on the right side of the bed, when it starts in earnest: The heaving rattle of her labored breathing, as though every exhale is arduous. After hours of listening to her unsettling breathing pattern, this one is markedly different. It is the breath of death. I grab both her hands, afraid to leave to get everyone because I don't want to leave her.

What do I say? What do you say when your mother is dying? What does she want?

I start mumbling The Lord's Prayer aloud. We're not a very religious family. My mother was raised Catholic, my father Congregationalist. When they married, my parents did so in an Episcopal church, which we attended until I was twelve and they left because they said they didn't like the internal politics of the place. They never joined another church. I married a Jewish man and we are raising our children in the Unitarian Universalist church while celebrating both Christian and Jewish holidays in our home.

I can't explain why The Lord's Prayer pops into my head and crosses my lips. This surprises me as I hear myself speak, as does what I start muttering next, "I forgive you. I forgive you. I forgive you. I forgive you."

And, as I'm saying these words, I actually do, I forgive our relationship, our periods of estrangement, the tension caused by our disagreements, the discord when I told her I would not be vacationing at the Cape with her that one year, the disappointment that I never became her best friend. I forgive it all. I hope she does too and that, somewhere inside her head she isn't cursing me out and wondering, "What the hell is she saying she forgives *me* for?"

Scott pokes his head into the room. He had fled earlier, unable to endure the rattling breathing pattern.

"It's time!" I stage-whisper. "Get them."

My father and brother run into the room while Scott and my sister-in-law linger, just out of view of my mother. Sean sits on the left side of Mom's bed. Dad stands beside him and strokes her head. They utter words of love.

Then it is silent.

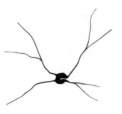

CHAPTER FIVE
The Downslide

I sleepwalk through the last weeks of the spring 2014 semester at the university. Dead woman walking. I remain mired in fog and phoniness. I pretend as if everything is fine and bury my actual feelings deep within me, refusing to show people how out-of-control everything feels right now.

I do not cry at my mother's bedside as she lay dying. (I save the crying for the solitary drive home, in gridlock, rush-hour Boston traffic, thankful for the stop-and-go as my vision is blurred by tears.) I do not cry at my mother's wake or at her funeral. Although I've spoken at both of my grandmothers' funerals and am comfortable speaking in public, I do not speak at Mom's funeral. I try to draft a eulogy at my desk but every draft I attempt comes off as defensive or self-deprecatingly devastating; the truth of what Mom was to me and me to her is complicated. Yes, I loved her. I know she loved me. However, our relationship stalled at an impasse that was never repaired and, in the immediate aftermath of her death, I'm unable to articulate my feelings because they're tangled up in a soup of emotion, not all of which are fit for a public eulogy. I abdicate the eulogy to Sean, who, although emotionally crushed, does a fine job. His relationship with her was much less fraught than mine.

I do not cry at the university as students ask why they can't find my name on the fall schedule or when students at the newspaper vigorously advocate for my reappointment as their adviser, and even write an editorial with veiled references to my job situation. I save that crying for the rides home from work, when I pass by that damned country club where I received the call about the brain mass, where I received the call about Mom. Every day, I feel the humiliation of being told, "We don't need you to continue teaching here next year" in every molecule but try to behave as though I don't.

I am thoroughly exhausted but write it off as the stress of the past six months. Meanwhile, that numbness that I experienced back in August 2012 when I was interviewing the band director, is roaring back to life on my left side. I'm torn between calling the neurologist, Dr. Sabine, the one who shamed me by suggesting that the symptoms were manifestations of my anxiety, and the consequences of *not* calling a doctor, which I just saw play out in front of my eyes in the person of my mother.

It's during a May bus ride from the Southborough middle school to a performance hall in Worcester when I make the decision to seek the opinion of a different neurologist, someone who specializes in multiple sclerosis. I talk it over with Jamie Clark, the band director who I was interviewing when I first experienced the numbness, who is now getting really antsy about the book I'm supposed to be writing about the year he and his Big Band spent mourning the loss of one of their bandmates. I haven't been working on that book. At all. The piles of notebooks filled with interviews and jazz band observations I made between September 2012 through June 2013 sit, forlorn, ignored in my home office. The several books on jazz and music education, likewise remain untouched. It all seems too much right now. I've spent the last several months dealing with Mom's illness, teaching at the university, and advising the student journalists. With the onset of this new fatigue that's impinging on my ability to just down a venti café latte and push through, I simply cannot muster the energy. I'm procrastinating on sitting down to write until summer break, after my time at the university comes to a permanent end.

Jamie doesn't bring up the fact that it's taking me a long time to write the first draft of the book, even though I stopped shadowing the group a year ago and have nothing tangible to show for it. He knows what's been going on. I am grateful that he is giving me the space I need to write the kind of book I want to write, one that will honor the compassionate teaching and guidance he provided his students, including Jonah. A lot of people—the kids who were in the Big Band during the year I followed them, all the band parents with whom I spoke, the Green family, people in the town of Southborough who were shaken by Eric Green's death—are counting on this book to be good. I feel the pressure in a distinct, tactile way even as swaths of my flesh seem to be going numb. I need to be in the right headspace, to allow myself to tap into my own authentic emotions, my own sense of ache in order to write about the students with any degree of credibility. It's a sacred place in which I simply cannot dwell, at least at this moment.

During the bus ride to Worcester, where I'm serving as one of the parent chaperones accompanying Casey's seventh and eighth grade concert band to their performance at Mechanics Hall, Jamie asks me how I'm faring, two months since my mom's death. With most people, I usually offer a bland, nondescript response to such an open-ended inquiry. But with Jamie, I've formed a bond of genuineness. In response to the extremely personal questions I have been asking him for over a year, he has told me he wants to learn about me too. Against my journalistic judgment, I let him know me. I let him become my friend.

"I think the symptoms are coming back," I confess, with no need to elaborate on what I mean by "the symptoms." His kind and concerned face is partially obscured by the hump of the moss green bus seat so I cannot assess his reaction. "I think I need to get another MRI."

"Maybe it's just the stress of everything," he suggests hopefully. He's an optimist at heart. He wants to believe I'm just stressed out. I wish I could believe him. I used to be an optimist. I'm not anymore.

⌒

Half of Mom has been buried, interred here, in a small, rural cemetery made of hills, ridges, and trees in the western Massachusetts town in which I grew up, the town in which Dad has resided for all but five years of his life. The remainder of her ashes will be laid to rest at a Wellfleet beach some time to be determined later. A tiny plaque has already been placed to mark the spot when we arrive: my family of five, Sean's family of five, Dad, and a smattering of other family members and friends of my parents, including my mother's brother from Philly. When Mom died in March, the ground here was too hard, too frozen to bury her. Now that it is May, it has thawed sufficiently for this ceremony.

I give each of my mother's six grandchildren, along with her two youngest nephews, a pink rose each. After the priest my father has asked to say a few prayers does his thing, the children form a solemn line and carefully place their flower atop the plaque. I distribute the remaining flowers to family and friends to do the same. My father's best friend Lenny and his wife Mary Jane distribute clear plastic wine glasses to the adults. Lenny—who, as a liquor salesman had my mother as a client—holds a fine specimen of vino aloft and makes a toast to Judy, the Wine Mother.

After the short service and everyone heads back to their vehicles, Dad appears behind my car. Acting as though he's handling illicit drugs, he shoves a box containing the other half of Mom inside something called a water urn (a supposedly biodegradable container with which you can deposit a loved one's ashes into a body of water) into my hands. One of the funeral home staffers gives it to Dad, who treats it like a hot potato, and hands it to me. He wants me to put it into the back of my SUV.

"Why Dad? Why do you want us to take this?"

He never answers my question, just walks away, frazzled. I pass the box to Scott, as both my father and I are unwilling or unable to handle what's inside.

The assorted mourners have lunch at Dad's favorite Italian restaurant, the place where nearly all the distinctive, rectangular-shaped pizzas of my childhood were prepared. Listening to the laughter and chatter emanating from the packed private room, I'm certain the other patrons wouldn't think we are there after interring someone's ashes. The mood sounds light. Like a lot of things I'm noticing these days, it's just an illusion.

⊷

The month of June 2014 begins with news that my nearly eighty-year-old mother-in-law has an abdominal aneurysm for which she has decided to blow off medical advice and decline the recommended surgery. It's a ticking time bomb in her belly.

Within the same week, Scott and I learn that she also fell on a sidewalk and badly banged herself up. The only reason we know this is because Scott's cousin stopped by her apartment and called Scott later to fill him in. She is reluctant to tell Scott what is happening and tends to keep health issues close to the vest.

A few hours later, I learn from my father's brother Larry that Dad fell down the porch stairs at my parents' house at three-thirty in the morning while letting his dog out, subsequently injuring his arm and shoulder as well as seriously bruising his face.

I'm starting to wonder whether someone, somewhere, has voodoo dolls of family members.

My sixty-seven-year-old father is falling apart. He shows up to a barbecue at Sean's house with a Gorbechev-like scab across the thinning brown and gray hair on the top of his head. He says he scraped it on a bathroom cabinet door in the middle of the night. The true story behind that scab is anyone's guess, as are the tales behind the array of cuts and scrapes across his legs, arms, and face. They can't all be from that one fall when he let the dog outside at three-thirty in the morning.

Dad walks hunched over, haltingly, in obvious pain (bad knees, one failed knee replacement later). His six-foot frame is involuntarily shaking. He is not eating much these days. He's not sleeping at all, at least not at night. (He's developing the sleeping habits of a college student, sleeping during the day, staying awake at night.) He doesn't seem to care about taking care of himself or the house which Mom so painstakingly decorated with finds from craft fairs and galleries.

In the months after Mom died, when I visit the house—the two-bedroom Cape my parents bought in the mid-1970s, where every inch is now decorated by and filled with things my mother acquired—it's as if its appearance mirrors the way the inside of Dad's head feels. Piles of papers cover the kitchen table. The gift basket of gourmet food Scott and I gave my parents for Christmas is still on the kitchen counter. Every surface is covered with something. His bed is unmade, and it looks like the sheets haven't been changed in a very long time. There's hardly any food in the fridge and what is there is rotting.

I rue the day he decided to retire—Sean, Mom, and I all told him it was a bad idea—because now he has an empty house and nothing to do all day but perseverate about the last few months. Sean and I have spoken with him about getting some grief counseling.

"There's no shame in seeing someone Dad," I tell him during a planned sit-down in Sean's living room during the early summer barbecue. "I see a therapist for my anxiety. It's for your mental health. That's as important as your physical health."

"I don't need it," Dad says, echoing the refrain he repeatedly told hospital staffers when they offered up services for the newly bereaved, "I have a strong family. I don't need it."

"But Dad, we aren't therapists," Sean says. "We're not equipped to help you. Therapists can."

I chime in: "And support groups with people who've lost spouses to cancer will understand what you're going through better than we can. We haven't lost our spouses. We lost our mom. It's different. They could help. Maybe could just listen."

But he won't. Stubborn Irishman.

⤶

Dr. Walker is the head of the multiple sclerosis unit at a Boston hospital. I carefully research him before booking an appointment because I don't want to replicate what happened with Dr. Sabine when he treated me as though my numbness leapt directly out of my imagination. Now that the symptoms I experienced two years ago have returned and new ones are appearing, I know I need to work fast. The numbness along my left leg is again spreading, climbing up the left side of my torso to my chest so that side of my body registers only a dull touch. At night, my legs are starting to spasm and jerk ever-so-slightly, demanding that I stretch them out. Even more worrisome is another new symptom: the tingling and radiating heat sensation—like when an extremity that has fallen asleep starts waking up—that periodically dances beneath the flesh of my left side. After Googling these symptoms, I am worried all signs point to MS.

To keep myself busy in the hours before my June neurological appointment, I complete online applications for part-time positions at local universities and colleges to teach writing or journalism. I am determined that, despite everything that's happening, I will move forward. Once those applications are complete, Scott and I drive to Boston to meet the new neurologist, a tall but soft-spoken man in his mid-forties, with professorial-looking glasses, salt-and-pepper hair and a goatee. When my name is called, I pointedly ask the salt-and-pepper haired, goateed Scott not to come into the examining room with me. I do not want his presence to undermine my credibility with this guy like it did with Dr. Sabine. I do not want to appear weak or in any way incapable of discussing what has been going on.

Once inside the exam room, I lay out my situation quite plainly, with brutal honesty, bearing in mind that the mention of anxiety treatment could, to some, present a bright red flag, as could my mother's untimely death at age sixty-five, plus the non-renewal of my teaching contract. I do not mention my father's disintegration, which just seems like overkill.

Dr. Walker appears to be listening intently, with no judgment, at least none that I can detect. In a letter he writes to my primary care physician later, he indicates he's taking my concerns seriously. "She does have slightly decreased range rapid alternative movements on the left arm," he writes. "Light touch, vibration, temperature and pinprick are all normal except for decreased pin in the whole left leg, the torso mainly in the back, less in the front. She has decreased temperature sensation in the left upper and lower extremities." He orders a new MRI and tells me he wants to see me in four months.

As I stand up to leave, he walks me to the doorway. Dr. Walker has a glossy white folder in his hands. He looks like he's going to hand it to me. But he doesn't. I notice that it's a folder for newly diagnosed MS patients. He reiterates that I only have one lesion, not multiple lesions, that I do not yet qualify for the official definition of multiple sclerosis, but still,

MEREDITH O'BRIEN

58

he hesitates. Like he knows something I don't and he's weighing whether to share it.

He tells me later that when he's diagnosing patients he likes to "set them up," lay the groundwork for what's likely to happen next, saying things like, "There's a high probability of MS," or "we'll just watch closely and see."

Before I leave, Dr. Walker smiles, purses his lips, and hands me the folder.

⌣

It's late June when Dad himself is admitted to the hospital, the same one where my mother went during her Emergency Room trip and for her uterine surgery last fall. In fact, my father is brought to the exact same ER patient bay in which my mother initially resided, something I inform the ER nurses to change immediately after Dad mentions it to me.

Uncle Larry had called me earlier on that steamy afternoon to tell me Dad's primary care physician, who had run a panel of blood tests, urged Dad to go to the hospital because his liver function is seriously impaired. Additionally, Dad is having even more difficulty walking and is incredibly weak.

This is a complete shitshow, I text a friend, absolutely incredulous that I'm heading back to the hospital so quickly to care for another parent.

Scott leaves work early in the eastern part of the state and takes me on the hour-and-a-half drive to the hospital in western Massachusetts. I'm too shaken up by this news to drive. When we get there, Uncle Larry looks relieved because now he can go home. He's spent hours with Dad at the hospital already.

My six-foot-tall father is diminished, in body, in spirit. I try not to look shocked when I see him, try to conceal the question that has been haunting my dreams, in between reliving my mother's death scene repeatedly every night, causing me to wake with a tumultuous gastrointestinal system.

Am I going to lose both parents in the same year? I ask myself as I take in the whole scene.

He looks as though he's been beaten. And he has. By life. By loss. By loneliness. This recently-retired liquor salesman, the one with the contagious sense of humor and a funny story always at the ready, the guy in the group who's most likely to give you a nickname, the one who loves books, old movies, dogs, politics, cooking, and the Red Sox ... well, he doesn't know what to do with himself now that his wife of forty-five years is no longer beside him. I have no idea what to do to help him.

~

Altogether, Dad spends five days in the hospital. On the second-to-last day, Sean's eight-year-old son is rushed to a Boston hospital with what doctors believe is acute pancreatitis. Dad's care is left up to me, as Sean leaves the western Massachusetts hospital to go to a Boston one. When I get home that night, Sean's other two sons—ages ten and four—are staying the night at my house, along with Dad's geriatric poodle Kelly. Gallows humor runs rampant through the text messages I exchange with Sean and a couple of friends whose responses to the new news are usually along the lines of, "Seriously?!"

Once Sean's son is stable and is eventually released from the hospital, the two of us work to persuade Dad to go from the hospital to a rehab facility in eastern Massachusetts, closer to both of us so we can see him every day during his physical rehabilitation. Scott and I volunteer to drive Dad to the rehab facility. However, we should have done our homework beforehand. The facility to which he is transferred is, in a word: horrendous. It smells like puke and ripe feet. There are strange stains on the hallway carpet. Before entering the building, we witness an adult daughter of a resident smearing Vick's

VapoRub across her mother's upper lip. "It's the only way to deal with the smell," she says, seemingly resigned to her mother's lot. Within minutes of bringing Dad's wheelchair into the facility we realize the place is a disaster. Scott and I quickly confer in the hallway, which reeks to the point where I'm covering my face with my hands and trying not to retch. There is no way Dad is staying here, we decide. Scott takes charge and tells Dad to get back into the wheelchair and brings him to the car again. We will find another facility in which he will recuperate, we tell the staffers who chase out the door asking us why we are leaving.

Our timing. It sucks. So badly.

Staff at rehabilitation facilities and insurance companies are on their July 4 breaks. Getting my father transferred to a clean facility that does not require the application of a menthol gel to kill the smell, takes days of phone calls and exasperation and red tape so, for the time being, Dad is staying at our house. Problem is, he can't really walk. He isn't fully functioning. He keeps falling down. He can't make it up the stairs to the bedrooms in our Colonial, so we set him up in the family room, the same room where my mother, months earlier, slept when she was dying from cancer. I sleep in the adjacent sunroom so I can hear any time Dad rolls around or gets up. I am a watchdog. I sleep very little as he rolls around restlessly, falls off the sofa upon which he insists on sleeping, instead of a bed which we've offered to set up in the room.

When he wakes up on our sofa the first morning after being released from the hospital, he sees Jonah and Casey and gets confused. "Hey kids, where's your grandma?" he asks them.

↩

I make an absolute nuisance of myself. But for once, the woman who hates bothering others, hates inconveniencing them, hates causing a stink of any kind, does not care. I am calling Dr. Walker's office repeatedly.

"Do you have my MRI results yet? ... Well can you tell me when you'll have them? I'm leaving for a ten-day-trip to California from July 15 through the 26th. I want to get the results before I leave."

I speak with the same office manager several times. Each time, my pleas get more desperate. I do not want to leave on this much-needed family vacation to the west coast without learning the results of the new MRI I had at Dr. Walker's behest.

⌇

Dad is finally situated at a rehab facility nearby. Unlike the last place, I do not see any dead bugs lying around his room. There is no offensive smell. His roommate is a senior citizen who likes to hang out in the community room and doesn't have an odorific jar of pickles next to his bed like his previous would-be roommate did. The staff members at the new place are genial and accommodating. Maybe they can reach Dad, break through his impenetrable, shell of mourning. Although my father looks lost and painfully vulnerable, I feel, for the first time since Mom died, that he is safe, unbearably heartbroken, but safe.

Back at my house, Dad's dog Kelly is not getting along with my dog Max. Kelly is a black, fifteen-pound, hyper-yappy, aged, pure-bred, skittish poodle. Max is a chill, tan, thirty-pound rescue mutt who just wants to hang and eat food. Kelly, however, wants to screw, or at least pretend to as the neutered dog frequently tries to mount Max. Taller than Max due to his long, thin legs, Kelly also takes to urinating on Max's head. It's no surprise when Max starts spending a lot of time holed up in Abbey's bedroom just to get away from his horny stalker.

Daily life seems as if it has emerged from a darkly comedic independent film. The kids are very helpful in the wake of all this chaos, walking Max and Kelly around the neighborhood, accompanying me to visit my father at the rehab center, trying to cheer him up by bringing him snacks, and reading material. Abbey, Jonah, and Casey are bearing up reasonably well, adeptly playing the roles of court jesters just to see Grandpa's white whiskers rise with a meek smile that I suspect is fake. They just want him to be happy.

I remain determined that, despite Dad's rehab stay, my family of five will still go on our trip to California. A month after Mom died, I decided we needed a vacation far away from our lives. I felt compelled to put three thousand miles between us and the hideousness of the past few months. I wanted to try something different. I picked LA. I wanted to sit in the LA sun, swim in the Pacific Ocean, and do all the touristy things one does when in Hollywood, the place of stars and dreams. My children—who, at ages fifteen, fifteen, and twelve, bore witness to their grandmother's rapid decline on our family room sofa and in the hospital, attended her wake and funeral, saw my sadness over my work situation, and also observed the swift deterioration of their grandfather's health—are absolutely in need of some frivolity. Scott, who quietly shoulders the burden of planning the trip, as well as trying to deal with his wife's growing emotional tumult, takes care of all the travel arrangements. He books us a rental unit, gets us reservations for baseball and soccer games, and tours of famous LA venues. When I hand off my father's care—along with custody of the horny hound—to Sean and his wife Lisa, I am gleeful. I am free, free from the drama of death, of work, or mourning ... at least for ten days.

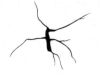

CHAPTER SIX

Partner in Crime

He appeared suddenly from around the corner of the brick wall behind which I was hiding. His right hand was aloft above his head. A small snowball sat in his palm, like a baseball about to go barreling from the pitcher's hand into the catcher's mitt. I was startled. I didn't see him approaching as I sought cover from the nighttime snowball fight in November 1987 in the center of the University of Massachusetts' cluster of seven-story dorm buildings on Orchard Hill. But there he was, his dark eyes brimming with mischief, his even darker, thick hair dusted with snow, his puffy gray winter jacket crinkled in concert with his movement.

He's going to kiss me, I thought. It wasn't an unreasonable thought. Ever since the sophomore engineering major visited my dorm room on Grayson Hall's third floor to hit on my roommate—but, instead, wound up arguing with me about the re-flagging of Kuwaiti ships with U.S. flags—an ember had been smoldering, ignited during that debate as I labored over my freshman political science paper. It flickered during the group activities with the girls on my floor and the boys from his. I was dating someone else. Someone from high school. I wasn't looking for anybody new. But, in reality, I was, I just didn't realize it. I was looking for him.

I arched my eyebrows and stared back at him.

He's not going to hit me with that snowball. He's going to kiss me.

The moment felt like it was moving in slow-motion. We locked eyes. I sharply drew in a quick breath. He leaned toward me, but not to go for a kiss, to get traction on the snow before pivoting in another direction to drill one of his floormates with the snowball.

We started dating a few months later, eight days after he bought long stem roses for the women in our group of friends for Valentine's Day. At first, I felt a twinge of jealousy as I saw him give a red rose to female after female, a move that annoyed the guys from the second floor who felt showed up by his display of chivalry.

Am I just one of the crowd? I asked myself.

After he gave my roommate a flower, he handed me one too, but mine was accompanied by a card, a sweet one, something no one else got. It had a fluffy dog on it. Soon, I found myself on the telephone with my long-distance boyfriend, with whom I'd been corresponding (old school, via handwritten, snail-mailed letters), and we decided to see other people. After I attended a formal spring dance at the long-distance guy's school in early 1988, we amicably decided to part ways. At age eighteen (almost nineteen), I decided to date only Scott, who was almost twenty and who hadn't been in a relationship that lasted longer than two months.

⌐

It was a loud party. I was surprised no one had called the cops yet. Scott and his three roommates, all senior engineering majors, had two kegs of cheap beer on the balcony of their two-bedroom apartment and were charging party-goers a few bucks a piece to help defray the costs. The place was packed. Whatever music that was blaring from the CD player—REM, Billy Idol, The Beatles, The Stones—was drowned out by the sound of drunk or nearly-drunk college kids.

As the party was starting to wind down in the wee hours

of the morning, I was in the kitchen with a friend, sitting at the small, crumb-covered kitchen table (one that would later take up residence in my first post-college apartment). I had a plastic cup in my hand. I was buzzed, buzzed in a way that made me act like I had more courage than I actually possessed when I was sober. Then this guy—an engineering major with whom Scott had a few classes, someone I didn't know but was a friend of a friend—entered the kitchen. He butted into the conversation I was having with my friend about the George H.W. Bush administration. The guy had a boozy look in his eyes and didn't like what he heard. He lobbed some aggressive, verbal counterpunches to fiercely rebut mine.

Filled with youthful brio, I regularly penned extremely idealistic and liberal columns for the student newspaper, of which I would, in my senior year, become editor-in-chief. I liked the back-and-forth exchange of ideas—that was one of the first things Scott and I did together, debate politics—but I didn't like debating anyone who was angry-drunk or who was a raging sexist. When the drunk guy's arguments mutated into a misogynistic salvo of insults, liquid courage propelled me to yell loudly and uncharacteristically, "Scott! Get this fucking asshole out of here!"

Scott, as buzzed as everyone else, was in the living room with his roommates. He muttered, "Here we go." This drunk guy and his friends had a reputation for getting loaded at parties and wrecking stuff. The thinly-built Scott was not a fighter. It was not in his nature. While he was someone who wanted to fix every problem he saw, he tended to be more of a deliberative, keep-one's-emotions-in-check kind of person. But tonight, he was that guy, the one who took on the inebriated. He surprised the drunk guy, who had many pounds and a couple inches on him. Scott put his hands, palm-forward, on the drunk guy's chest, pushed him through the galley kitchen, and stopped pushing when they ran out of room and the guy's back was up against the wall next to the front door. The people in the room froze. Scott's three roommates, also relatively thin and not the fighting type either, girded themselves. They were worried. They were preparing to back up Scott who was backing me up, the mouthy junior journalism and political science major who was sitting at the kitchen table, holding the plastic cup of beer, unaware of how the atmosphere in the apartment had shifted like quicksilver.

"It's time to leave," Scott said in the deepest booming tone he could make.

To everyone's surprise, the drunk guy said nothing in response. He was calmly escorted out of the apartment by his friends. No punches were thrown. Nothing got broken. Tension slowly leaked out of the room, like helium from a balloon. Scott downplayed the exchange as his roommates audibly exhaled. They weren't going to have to mix it up with experienced brawlers. From my perch on the kitchen chair, I felt a jolt of pleasure at having a protector put himself, his body, in between me and the danger, and we both emerged unscathed.

If only it worked that way with illnesses. If only we could fix everything and literally push diseases out the door.

⌒

It was a tradition brought to this Westfield, Mass. table all the way from Poland, from my maternal grandfather's family who immigrated to New England in the early 1900s. On Wigilia (we pronounced it va-LEE-ah), my parents, Sean, my mother's brother Ted, and I usually went to Gram and Pap's house for a traditional, meatless Christmas Eve dinner featuring pierogis, apple-rice casserole, and baked stuffed shrimp. Before eating, we took turns passing individual Christmas wafers—the oplatek, a larger version of a communion wafer—to the person sitting to our left. Each person broke off pieces of the wafer, ate the pieces, and wished the wafer owner good tidings for the coming year. In my family, the wishes were personalized, like wishing Sean good luck with his freshman year of college, or hoping Mom has a good year at the two wine shops she managed. On occasion, the wishing transformed into mini-interventions, like when Mom told her father everyone knew he was sneaking cigarettes in the backyard and wished he would stop. After she shared her wishes, everyone else added being smoke-free into their hopes for my grandfather.

Up until this year, 1991, people not directly related to the family did not attend our Christmas Eve dinner. However, Scott and I were now living together, a fact all the adults at the table liked to pretend wasn't happening. I graduated from college in May and lived with my parents for a few months as I started my career as a newspaper reporter. In September, Scott and I found an apartment halfway between his workplace and mine. I informed my parents and grandparents we were moving in together and that the apartment had two bedrooms. We all silently stuck with the collective fiction that Scott and I occupied those separate bedrooms and my folks mostly withheld their disapproval of my decision. Despite my scandalous living situation—never mind the fact that he was Jewish and I was Protestant—Gram told me to bring him to Wigilia. I prepped him for potentially awkward situations, like people criticizing one another through passive-aggressive wafer wishes. I told him my mother and her brother liked to harass my grandfather about smoking and that they wanted him to sell his auto body shop. Mom also liked to make heavy-handed wishes about Sean and I getting along better, and about Sean helping more around the house. I had no idea what they would say to Scott, the guy who was living in sin with me.

As we sat down at the lace-and-transparent-plastic-sheet-covered dining room table, a Frank Sinatra Christmas album played on my grandparents' turntable. The smell of butter-saturated cheese and sauerkraut pierogis tantalizingly lingered in the air. My grandfather's wafer was passed around first. Scott did not sound at all uncomfortable as he broke off small pieces and wished Pap health and another good year with his business. When my wafer started making its way around the table, Gram wished me continued success with my journalism career, as did my uncle. Sean muttered something about me doing "good work," then passed my wafer to my father. It went to my mother, then to my grandfather, then, eventually, to Scott, who pushed his chair back, dropped to his right knee, and proposed to me. In a strange domino-like effect, I started crying, followed by my grandmother, and my mother. My father abruptly got up from the table and fled to the adjacent kitchen, sobbing, crestfallen that his little girl was going to get married. Even my normally emotionally-withholding grandfather's eyes teared up. My brother's and uncle's eyes remained dry. They were eager to get on with it and dive into those pierogis and that shrimp.

After the waterworks, it dawned on my uncle that I never actually said, "Yes" to the proposal.

"Oh, she said, 'Yes!' She said, 'Yes!'" Gram blurted. Tears appeared anew as they dripped into Gram's champagne flute that my mother had filled.

⤙

We married on Halloween night in 1992 in an historic New England meeting house in my hometown, with a Jewish cantor and an Episcopal minister officiating. We were not big Halloween fans, mind you. October 31 just happened to be the only Saturday evening in the fall that was available at the meeting house. We wanted to marry in the fall because it was so picturesque in this collection of colonial-era buildings at Storrowton Village. We needed a Saturday night because some of Scott's more Orthodox relatives wouldn't attend a Friday evening or Saturday daytime service. Halloween night was open, so we booked it.

As my bridesmaids and I dressed for the ceremony in the

second floor of the colonial-era Potter house, directly across from the meeting house, the piped-in sounds of cackling witches and scary sound effects playing for those attending Halloween events in other parts of Storrowton Village, added a bit of theater to the event. I tried not to read it as an ominous sign.

Hours later, during the reception inside the Storrowton Tavern Carriage House across the courtyard from the meeting house, the DJ asked everybody to clear the dance floor. Off to the right side of the room, Scott and the groomsmen appeared with gel-slicked hair, powdered faces, and plastic vampire teeth crammed in their mouths. Scott was the only one wearing a cape. "Thriller" boomed through the speakers. The guys started to dance rather stiffly until their dates accompanied them on the dance floor. When I reached Scott's side, he attempted to playfully bite my neck, way before *Twilight* was a thing. Surprised, I pulled my neck away and sort of playfully, sort of not, shoved him back, uneasy, even on my wedding day, of becoming a spectacle.

⌇

In the summer of 1997, Scott found me in our newly-rented basement apartment in Marlborough, Mass. We recently moved back to Massachusetts after having lived in the Washington, D.C. area for several years so I could attend graduate school and work at a journalism think-tank. I resumed teaching journalism part-time at a university and was working as a freelance writer. I was also trying to get pregnant. It was time. But my body was not cooperating. Hadn't been for months. I'd been trying to get pregnant since 1996 with no luck. After enduring several invasive and embarrassing tests, we underwent a half-dozen rounds of infertility treatments, with me taking a lot of fertility medication, one which required injections which Scott gave me because I was too chicken to give them to myself. When Scott came home from work on that summer evening, I was sitting in the darkened apartment, and crying. I had just found out that another attempt had failed.

He shook his head and wrapped me in an embrace. There wasn't much more he could do to help us get through this, to shove the uncertainty of whether we'd ever have children aside, like he did with that drug guy at the keg party. The infertility, however, was a much more formidable opponent than an inebriated college student. He felt like a helpless witness, a thwarted problem-solver who could not make it better.

We were going to start in vitro fertilization at the beginning of the new year but with the chances of success low, I decided I didn't want to teach part-time and be a freelance writer who worked from home any longer. I needed to get out of the apartment, away from the reminders of my disappointment, my failure to start a family while friends and family members seemingly got pregnant with ease. I started looking for a full-time job. The week I was slated to start my new job as a newspaper reporter in Boston, in January 1998, I learn I'm pregnant. With twins. Nothing, I learn, ever works out the way I think it will.

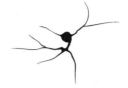

CHAPTER SEVEN
A Hollywood Storybook

It's early on a mid-July 2014 morning and still dark, when I drag myself out of bed, throw on clothes, and quickly gulp down a cup of coffee. We have a seven-twenty-five a.m. flight from Logan Airport in Boston to LAX in Los Angeles and, despite our sleepiness, we are all excited. Scott and the kids have never been to LA. The last time I went I was twelve and attending my maternal great-grandparents' sixtieth wedding anniversary. After we check our bags with the skycap outside the airport, we see Hilary Knight, a forward for the silver-medal-winning USA women's hockey team. She's on her way to the ESPYs in LA. My sports aficionado daughter Abbey recognizes her immediately and gets Scott to approach the Olympic athlete to ask if she'd pose for a photo with her young fan.

"Do you want to wear my medal?" Knight asks fifteen-year-old Abbey, extracting the silver from a long sock tucked inside her carry-on bag.

"Yes!" Abbey says without hesitation, thrilled as the hockey star lowers the medal over the rising high school sophomore's neck as if she was standing atop a podium.

After a few girl-power photos, Knight invites Jonah and Casey to join them. I tweet out the photo of the four of them, making sure to tag Knight—a news junkie, I'm kind of obsessive about Twitter—and grab hard onto the idea that this is going to be charmed adventure to the west coast. The silver medal is a sign, a promise of shimmering waters, of sunlight cutting through palm trees, of serenity. A new beginning.

Many hours later after a cross-continental flight, we are pulling our rental SUV up to the classic, stucco-covered California bungalow we've rented on 4th Street in Santa Monica which is lined with palm trees. We chuck our belongings into our respective bedrooms then head out on foot to explore. We walk the pedestrian-friendly Third Street Promenade, meander through Palisades Park on Ocean Avenue, and dip our feet in the Pacific Ocean en route to the Santa Monica Pier. Hours later, after dark, we crash into our beds when we return to the house, our bodies still on East Coast time, our heads slowly easing into a California state of mind.

I'm drinking coffee the following morning, still a little blurry-headed with jet lag when my cell rings. It's Dr. Walker. He has my MRI results.

"Hold on Dr. Walker," I say, scanning the glass kitchen table for something on which I can jot notes. The closest thing I can find is my paperback copy of Meg Wolitzer's *The Interestings* which I'd been reading on the airplane. I flip to the last blank page and motion to Scott to toss me a pen. He throws me a red one. Red. The color of emergencies. Danger. Warning.

"I need you to come in right away," Dr. Walker says urgently.

I hold my tongue. Because I'm pissed. I had repeatedly called his office and begged for the results before I left on a ten-day trip to California. I'd told his staff I was going away. "I am in Los Angeles on vacation."

There's a pause on the other end. Dr. Walker is weighing his words. I am sitting, thousands of miles away, and can imagine him pursing his lips, the way he did when he was trying to decide whether to hand me a brochure about MS.

"I will make an appointment to come to see you as soon as I get home," I say. "What did the results say?"

"There is a change in your MRI but it's not overwhelmingly so."

I do not understand. *What does a "not overwhelmingly so"*
change mean?

He unpacks the results: "It looks like there are new changes." I go into reporter mode and write down phrases and details inside the book. Dr. Walker says I have three new brain lesions, including one in the area that connects the two hemispheres of the brain, next to my formerly lone lesion on the brainstem/C-spine area. One of the lesions has "enhancement," he says, meaning, at the time I had the MRI, two weeks prior, the area around that disease-damaged nerve was inflamed.

Medical records I read later report that the following were found in my brain:

A 9 x 6 mm lesion in the splenium of the corpus callosum to the left of the midline

A 9 mm lesion on the left cerebellum

An ill-defined lesion in the anterior aspect of the cord

A 10 mm hyperintensity in the cervical spinal cord, central/anterior spinal cord (This was the original lesion.)

Perhaps I am not fully awake yet or that the caffeine hasn't properly hit my system, but I never ask Dr. Walker *the* question: *Do I have multiple sclerosis?* Maybe he thinks it's now obvious that I do, considering we're talking multiple lesions, but Dr. Walker never says it definitively during the phone call. How can this escape my notice? Maybe I don't want to see what's nakedly obvious, just like Mom didn't want to acknowledge she was dying. Maybe I'm just plain stunned.

Meanwhile, Dr. Walker continues in that even-keeled tone of his. He wants to speak with the radiologists who read the MRI and see me in his office when I get back to Massachusetts. He wants me to have another MRI as soon as possible.

For someone who prides herself on researching everything to death, on asking the hard questions of people I interview, I am speechless. I fail to ask the right questions. I fail to ask *any* questions other than whether he had the MRI results. I don't even pull out my smartphone, from which I'd been tweeting and Instagramming photos of Santa Monica to my social media followers, to see for myself what this new information means.

I hang up the phone and place it softly on the glass table. Scott, who has been listening and reading what I wrote down in the book, looks really scared.

"Well," I say, "there's nothing I can do about this now. I wish he had called before I left."

Scott doesn't ask whether Dr. Walker said I have MS. We're both stuck on the fact that I have lesions in my brain and spine. Lesions. *Multiple*. That weren't there two years ago. At least one of which was or is still actively inflamed. Who knows how many are inflamed now, weeks later? What having an inflamed lesion means I don't quite understand on that California morning. And I don't look it up. I don't want to. I'm here for that new beginning I've promised everyone, including myself.

My coffee grows cold and my mind goes blank. Context eludes me. Scott rises from his chair on the other side of the table and hugs me. We don't say a whole lot, which is very unusual for us. We will not tell the kids, at least not yet. We don't really know what this means. In reality, we do know, deep down inside, but we don't really want to accept it. Not right now.

⟿

As our tour cart passes what was once downtown Stars Hollow, Conn. from the TV show *Gilmore Girls*, a drama about the lives of a highly-caffeinated mother and daughter duo, I squeeze Abbey's hand. This TV show is meaningful to us, as she sees herself as the studious Rory and me as talkative, coffee-obsessed Lorelai. Although the set is currently being used for another TV show, the bones of the fictional Connecticut town are still there. We can see them from inside our

Warner Brothers Studio cart. A little while later, Abbey is the one who squeezes my hand as we walk around the set for *The Fosters*, a currently-filming TV show about two moms raising a family of adopted children. We traipse through the kitchen, characters' bedrooms, and the back yard where many heartfelt conversations between the fictional family members take place. Later, all five of my family members are enthralled by the collection of Harry Potter costumes and props the studio has on hand: Death Eater costumes, Gringotts' goblins, Dobby the elf, Tom Riddle's diary. Years earlier, Scott and I read nearly the entire Potter series aloud to Casey and we've collectively watched all of the films multiple times together. Jonah and Casey, however, are most impressed with an actual Batmobile from one of the many *Batman* films, and with using the prop fire extinguishers, two-by-fours, and shovels to play-fight. We are marinating ourselves in fiction, in the land of make-believe. It feels safe, even with the Death Eaters.

We take in the sweeping views from the Griffith Observatory, a locale made famous by many Hollywood productions, notably *A Rebel Without a Cause*. Despite the heat and blazing afternoon sunshine, we walk the adjacent Griffith Park grounds. I walk briskly, with determination, trying to find my son Jonah, who has taken off down one of the paths. Normally, I'm not a hiking kind of person. I would never be a Cheryl Strayed-*Wild* adventurer. I'm more of a movie-watcher, restaurant-goer, relax-on-the-beach, take-in-a-baseball-game or curl-up-with-a-good-book kind of gal. Yet I feel compelled to take off along a path, my "Boston Strong" Red Sox hat shielding my eyes from the sun, as I scale some steep areas while Scott, Abbey, and Casey, a rising eighth grader, horse around in the shade of a cluster of trees at the bottom of a hill. Rivulets of sweat start trickling down my neck and saturate the back of my sleeveless shirt. I realize I am stomping my feet as I climb rocky areas, leaving the easier paths untraveled. I start to feel light-headed and realize I need to cool off so I don't faint.

I hope that Jonah comes into view soon, I think.

⮑

Every day of our California sojourn features a little some-thing for everyone. One day as we're driving down the Pacific Coast Highway in our rental car—something Scott has always wanted to do—we make a stop at Malibu Seafood. The line to gain entry to what looks like a glorified shack, winds around the parking area in the midday sun. A little while and a lot of perspiration later, I enjoy my very first fish taco as we sweat at our picnic table overlooking the Pacific. We take Jonah, our resident drummer—he's a jazz and rock percussionist—to tour the DW drum showroom in Oxnard, north of Los Angeles. On another day, we hit a Santa Monica beach, just a short walk from our bungalow. I read *The Interestings* while Scott and the kids swim and body surf. There is no shade anywhere. We do not have an umbrella, but we've brought plenty of sunscreen to protect us from sunburns.

On yet another day, we perspire our way down the Holly-wood Walk of Fame, snap photos of one another fitting our hands and feet into celebrity imprints at Grauman's Chinese Theater, grab take-out from a local deli and walk to the Holly-wood Bowl where Scott has bought us tickets to see the Hollywood Bowl Orchestra play music from animated films. The performance will be emceed by comedic actor Jack Black. Our seats are far from the stage—in the last section—but they're in the first row of the last section, affording us plenty of leg room. Thankfully, the sun has finally set, rendering the sky a bubblegum pink. I take a photo and post it on Instagram. Everything feels so peaceful, calm. "Idyllic" comes to mind, an adjective that I don't typically use. We eat our food as the cheerful music plays and Jack Black provides lively commen-tary. Scott has planned this charmed trip to perfection. The music, the comfort food, the fact that we're all getting along so well transports me to a contented internal space. Things like MRI results are buried deep inside me; I refuse to think about them and sully this. I exhale, a deeply cleansing exhale, the kind you do at the end of your yoga practice when you're lying on your mat in an unburdened state. It feels like I'm living on a Hollywood set for a TV sitcom where a goofy but lovable family goes on a big trip.

Three pieces into the orchestra's performance, I feel a painful stinging sensation in the back of my head accompanied by immediate, urgent nausea, the kind of nausea you can't ignore. Thinking that perhaps there was some dairy in the take-out—even though we repeatedly told the folks at the deli that I have a dairy allergy—I head to the ladies' room thinking I'm having an allergic reaction.

I never return to my seat.

I spend the rest of the first half of the performance getting violently ill in the bathroom. Every time I think the nausea has passed and I slowly stand upright, my head throbs, I feel dizzy and start retching again. This is worse than any allergic reaction I've ever had.

Maybe it's food poisoning?

I hunch over in my sleeveless, blue cotton dress, lean my back against the stall door and my head toward the dirty floor. My arms are wrapped around my abdomen in a tight self-embrace. Restless and frustrated, I repeatedly attempt to leave the stall, to return to my life. I wash my hands, splash cold water on my face and join a worried-looking Scott who is pacing around outside the women's bathroom. We sit together on a bench and I attempt to reassure him. "I'm feeling a little better," I say, wishing I had the power to make it so. Thinking of our kids sitting alone in their seats, I tell him, "Let's go." But as soon as I start to walk, I have severe pain in my head and feel like I'm going to be sick again, so I race back into the bathroom. This happens several times. At intermission, Scott summons the kids and tells them we're going to leave because I'm too sick.

Leaving the Hollywood Bowl, mid-show, is no easy feat, particularly when you are on the top level of the Bowl and are walking in a stooped-over position while clutching your stomach. All five of us are able to descend only one level before I have to run into another women's bathroom and park myself inside a stall to vomit. My limbs feel weak as hell and I'm having trouble standing. I tell Abbey, who is outside the stall door and getting strange looks from the bathroom attendant for her lurking, that I cannot make it all the way out of the Bowl, never mind all the way back to the car, parked in a lot a mile away from the venue. Abbey runs outside and tells Scott, who asks a staff person for help. As if by magic, a wheelchair appears and whisks me away into a room deep within the bowels of the facility. I am unable to take a good look at the room because I am laser-focused on the painful burning in the back of my head, the fact that I cannot stop dry-heaving, and my intense dizziness.

Scott, our resident fixer, swings into action. He and Casey literally run all the way out of the facility, down the street and to the lot where we parked our SUV, while the silent and petrified Abbey and Jonah stand vigil outside the Hollywood Bowl first aid station, as I retch into a plastic bag, only I have nothing left in my stomach. I cannot be a mom right now and reassure them that everything will be okay because I am at war with my own body, wondering how to stop whatever is happening which, at this point, doesn't feel like any kind of allergic reaction or case of food poisoning I've ever had. (Plus no one else got ill from the food.) I just want to go back to our seats and enjoy the music that I faintly hear in the background. The Hollywood Bowl staff allows Scott to pull our rented vehicle into an emergency entrance/exit where someone on the medical staff delivers me, in my wheelchair, along with my two frightened teens.

By the time I am loaded into the car, we learn we have to wait because the post-performance fireworks display is happening. Inside the passenger seat, I sit with my forehead pressed into the passenger side dashboard and my knees pulled tightly into my chest. Feeling the deep *boom* of the fireworks blasts echoing inside me, I feel badly that the kids missed the rest of the performance and the fireworks and instead, got an exclusive gander at the first aid patient area.

To supplement my hazy memory of this evening, I asked Scott and the kids how they recalled this night.

From Abbey, who was fifteen at the time:

I was worried that you were so sick and that you had only eaten a little bit, that you should be taken to the hospital … You were just curled over the toilet. … I was spending my time running in and out of the stall, getting paper towels, putting cold water on them, putting them on your neck and forehead, and running back to Dad to give him updates.

… I remember finally, fifteen or twenty minutes later, you weren't getting any better, which was unusual because the allergies usually pass pretty quickly so then I think it was Dad who went to find someone. … When we realized you couldn't walk because you were too sick, when you couldn't move, you couldn't stand yourself up and support yourself, I think that's when Dad realized it was really bad. … I kept saying, "She needs to go to the hospital." I was kind of adamant about that, and I think Jonah and Casey kind of hooked onto that as well.

… We weren't allowed to go inside the room [in the Hollywood Bowl's medical triage room]. At the end of the show, they had fireworks and they were shooting them kind of near us. Dad was in the room with you. We were all freaked out because we didn't know where the fireworks were coming from, then someone warned us to be careful of the ashes landing in the area from the fireworks. And we were like, "Oh my God! What is happening?"

… We couldn't understand why Dad wasn't taking you to the hospital. It didn't make any sense to us. It was a mix of

confusion and just worry. ... It was weird because when you eat dairy, you throw up, you throw up everything, so I was just confused by that and confused by how long it was taking to pass, and I was thinking, "I hope she'll be okay by the morning."

From Jonah, who was also fifteen at the time:

Casey and I were standing outside the bathroom while Abbey was in there with you and you were having a really hard time throwing up. Then the security and emergency people showed up in the bathroom. And there were also some non-security people who were helping you out. They made a make-shift trash bin out of a cardboard box and put you in a wheelchair. ... I also remember that one of the emergency people was talking to Casey and I asking, "Is your mom in there? What happened?" We said, "We think she's having an allergic reaction." And then, they, like, took you away. The next thing I remember is we were down in this emergency room on the bottom floor while you were getting treatment.

... I also remember that they were setting off fireworks and we couldn't go out from the area. Ashes were coming down ... Casey was yelling at [Dad] for that because [Dad] kept poking his head out to see the fireworks.

... [Abbey and I] were outside the room you were in ... I didn't really know how serious it was, so I didn't know what to think.

Scott's perspective is a bit different from that of the kids, and rings loudly with second-guessing, regret, and explanation:

I could hear you in the bathroom, retching ... I thought the big issue had to do with you having had a dairy allergy reaction, that's what I assumed it was because we didn't know any better. I was thinking, "We need to get you to the car so we can get you home."

... Casey didn't want to stay [next to the triage room] so he went with me to get the car. We walked and ran. ... I was in a rush and [kept yelling], "Come on Casey! You need to keep up with me!"

Once he and Casey get the car and persuade Hollywood Bowl personnel to allow them to drive to the medical room, he is told we have to wait in the vehicle because they are about to set off fireworks for nearly thirty minutes. "I was anxious and impatient," Scott says of waiting for the fireworks show to end. "We felt trapped at the moment."

⌇

Against all logic and evidence to the contrary, I decide to call what happened at the Hollywood Bowl either food poisoning or some kind of unusual allergic reaction. I will not dwell on it. I will not research it on my phone. I will not even entertain the notion that it has anything to do with what Dr. Walker told me on the phone, or how he wanted me to see him immediately. I simply want that Hollywood Stars Hollow/*Gilmore Girls* life on the set, the kind of experience people think I am actually having when they look at my Facebook, Twitter, or Instagram feeds where I continue posting photos from our travels, photos of us smiling, laughing, living. There are no photos from inside the Hollywood Bowl first aid station or from one of the many bathroom stalls where I spent a considerable amount of time. I don't want to think about being ill. I want to see my children smile and laugh, do stupid stuff, and make memories.

Moving forward is complicated by the fact that I am severely weakened by "the incident." I feel very, very tired, and very, very guilty that I screwed up the entire Bowl experience by making us flee the premises as though we'd just committed a bank job. The melodrama, my having to physically lean on both my teens' shoulders in order to walk, scared them and scared me too. We traveled across the county to get away from the drama. Although all I really want to do is stay in bed someplace cool—the rented bungalow does not have air conditioning—I do not want to disappoint Scott, who poured so much time, money, and energy into planning this trip.

We have tickets for tonight's Los Angeles Angels game against the Seattle Mariners. Mike Trout, who would go on to be the American League's MVP and four-time All-Star, is slated to start at center field. He is hitting well too, averaging .311. I decide to join my family at this quotidian All-American event, a summer baseball game, like we're just a regular family on a regular vacation. The ballgame proceeds without incident as we sit in very comfortable outfield seats, which are much more comfortable than most of the seats in our beloved Fenway Park. We even get to enjoy a fireworks display after the game's last out, even though the home team lost, because that's what they do out here in Los Angeles after baseball games apparently, set off fireworks, win or lose. After a Red Sox game in Boston, they just play, "Dirty Water" as rowdy fans make for the exits, some busting out chants of "Yankees suck!" regardless of who the hometown played that night. Why? Because ... Boston. In California, however, everything's bigger, more Technicolor. Being able to see this fireworks display alleviates some of the guilt I feel about causing the family to miss the Hollywood Bowl fireworks. A teeny bit.

We cruise through the next several days in a state of cautious optimism, with me eating little and sleeping more. We visit the Ronald Reagan presidential library in Simi Valley, pose in front of Air Force One, see a replica of Reagan's Oval Office and a giant, graffiti-covered slab that was once part of the Berlin Wall. We leave our tainted Hollywood Bowl experience behind us and pretend as though it never happened. We are playing the roles of LA tourists, eating dinner at the Hard

Rock Café on Hollywood Boulevard and visiting Madame Tussauds' Hollywood where we take photos with wax statutes of George Clooney, Meryl Streep, Rihanna, J.Lo., and President Obama. We dine at the famous Smoke House restaurant in Burbank and gawk at a few celebs, buy food and flowers at the bountiful Santa Monica farmers' market, and attend an LA Galaxy-Manchester United soccer game at the Rose Bowl, thrilling my three soccer-crazed kids.

I am starting to get a little cocky. That Hollywood Bowl thing ... just an aberration. *Everything's fine*, I keep telling myself. Scott plays along.

Until the day when we're supposed to return to Boston.

That's when I wake up and experience that burning sensation in the back of my head again, feel light-headed and weak, and have the overwhelming urge to vomit. I crouch-walk to the bathroom, but have nothing other than stomach acid to throw up. I retch for a while, attempt to stand upright, get dizzy, see stars in my eyes, then sink to the floor again. I cannot blame this on anything food-related because I haven't eaten anything. Reality settles in hard. Now that we're heading home, I have to rip off the mask, the one I've been trying to present to the kids, that I've been presenting to myself, and look at the scary, ugly truth.

The doctor had wanted to see me right away.
Ten days ago.
There are new lesions in my brain
I am not okay.

Scott appears beside me. He wants to help but does not know what to do. We have to pack up and leave the house by eleven and I look as bad as I did at the Hollywood Bowl. Scott and Abbey maneuver me back to bed and allow me to lie there for as long as possible until they have to strip the bed and get me dressed. I lie there with my throbbing head and listen to my family pack up and clean the kitchen. I am so detached from it all, curled up in a ball while a fan blows warm air across my body. Scott and Abbey help me to the bathroom and Abbey gets me into the shower, but I am too dizzy to stand, too nauseous to not be curled up in a ball as I continue to violently retch. I sit on the shower floor, legs pulled up to my chest, as the water rolls down my head.

⮐

What was originally going to be a great opportunity—nearly a whole free day before our evening flight to Boston—is now a nightmare, particularly for Scott whose powers of fixing everything are being sorely tested. I am lying in a fetal position on top of a blanket in the shade of Palisades Park, gripping a plastic shopping bag tightly in my hands and occasionally dry-heaving into it. My family doesn't know what to do with me. The kids, who have been incredibly stoic, have no one to reassure them as Scott is focused completely on me. They only have one another and none of them know anything about the MRI results.

Since I have no first-hand memory of the rest of the day, Scott and the kids helped me fill in the gaps.

From Abbey:

> Dad and I were running around packing up the house, the food. I was packing up a bunch of your stuff. I know I helped you into the shower ... You sat down and I didn't really know what to do. When you got in there, you just needed to sit down. I knew something was really wrong. I knew it wasn't allergies. ... We had absolutely no information about anything. We were all just confused about why Dad wasn't taking you to the hospital or to see a doctor because he didn't seem to know what was going on. It was just kind of a scary thing and we didn't really know what to do. [Dad] was very tense, as he gets.

Scott remembers being focused on the immediate tasks at hand, packing the house, getting me to rest:

> *Everything had to be done with packing and you weren't in any shape to be able to do it. I remember barking at the kids a lot. I was yelling constantly ... I thought you would feel better. I thought it would go away. I didn't think any of this was MS ... I just figured you needed to rest.*

The stories they tell about what goes down at Palisades Park vary.

Abbey's version of events:

> *... I didn't think you were going to be able to fly because you couldn't stand up, you weren't with it. I almost thought you were going to lose consciousness at one point. You couldn't support yourself at all. You know right before you think someone is going to faint? Dad had been saying that if you can't fly, he was going to fly the three of us home.*

> *... When we were in the park, before Dad started making all the phone calls he was making to your doctor, Casey and I were asking what was going to happen and where we were going to stay. Dad kept saying, "I don't know! I don't know what we're going to do!" He was like, "You guys fly back!" ... I didn't like it. I know Jonah didn't like it. Jonah, I remember him saying, "No, we should all stay together." Casey and I agreed that it was best to stay together. ... I know Dad was not really thinking clearly because he was so worried about you. We tried not to argue with him.*

Jonah's perspective:

> *[When we were at the park I knew] you were having a really tough time and I didn't know what was going to happen with the plane because I knew you have a tough time on planes [because of motion sickness], and if you weren't feeling well, I didn't know if we were going to leave or not.*

... We were really worried about what was going to happen to you. If Dad wouldn't have wanted us to be with you guys at that point, it was because you were going through something. It seemed like Dad knew what you were going through and we didn't. Dad knew more than us. [I asked him what was going on] but he wouldn't tell me what was going on. He didn't seem like he knew what to do.

Scott remembers himself concentrating on what he can do next, how he can make plans to take care of everything:

You were semi-lucid and you basically just needed to lay down and you were almost passed out. At the time, I didn't know what to think. I didn't know what was going on. I didn't know what was wrong. I did underestimate how severe or serious your ailments were at the time ... My focus, right or wrong—and I can understand a lot of perspectives on this, that I should've called 9-1-1 and dealt with the ramifications— but I believed your ailment to be something temporary and you just needed to rest and you would recover and you would be okay. ... I just figured you needed to rest to be okay.

As for the idea of sending the kids on a plane to Massachusetts while he and I stayed behind in Los Angeles, Scott says:

I told the kids, "If Mom's not feeling well enough, we'll have to bring her to the hospital, and we'll have to send you on the plane." I didn't think they could stay, and we'd all hang around the hospital. Where would we stay? How would it work? I didn't know what to do. I had no support. ... The idea was that I'd send them on a plane, and I'd call someone to pick them up at the airport, to get 'em. They said, "Absolutely not. No! We're not doing that." So it was, "I gotta get you on a plane. How do we do that?" Maybe it was all wrong.

At lunchtime, Scott helps me into the driver's seat of our rental vehicle, which is parked next to Palisades Park with a view of the Pacific Ocean, and he turns on the AC. He walks the three kids to the Third Street Promenade, gives them a wad of cash and tells them to get something to eat. The whole time, they are asking one another if they think they'll have to fly home, cross-country, without their parents.

Here's Abbey's take on this:

> Dad was saying, "Okay, you guys need to go to get lunch."
>
> Casey said, "Johnny Rockets! Let's go there!"
>
> We said, "Fine." Dad gave me money. We sat down and we ate. Jonah and Casey had burgers. I had a tuna sandwich.
>
> We were talking, "Do you think we're going to have to fly back by ourselves? Do we think Mom is okay? Do you think Mom should go to the hospital? What do we think is happening?" ... I think we were all so worried that we didn't know what to do with ourselves.

They are, in fact, correct about their father. Wide-eyed and completely pale, Scott has no inkling of what to do. None of this is on the itinerary. His forty-five-year-old wife isn't supposed to be sick. Sure, she can be a bit nervous at times. She's obsessed with news and politics, the Red Sox and caffeine, yes, but sick and unable to function? No. He never imagined that, after nearly twenty-two years of marriage, he'd be running around Santa Monica to pick up medicine prescribed by a neurologist from thousands of miles away, leaving his wife slumped over and alone inside a rental car overlooking the Pacific Ocean, and pressing cash into his kids' hands so they'll go get lunch and buy himself some time to think.

As the kids return to the park, Scott is wrapping up a call Dr. Walker, telling him what is happening. The neurologist prescribes medicine that he thinks will help me get onto an airplane, a combination of anti-nausea medication and sedatives. Once I take them, Scott says, my nausea wanes but I am no more lucid than I was when we first got to the park: "You were actually feeling better, relatively speaking, your nausea was better, but you were so out of it. You were, essentially, drugged."

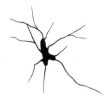

CHAPTER EIGHT
The Big One

I am lucky that the Ebola crisis has not yet arrived here in America yet because there is no way I would have been allowed to board a commercial airline in my condition: Glassy-eyed, unsteady, needing to lean on something or someone in order to remain upright as I make my way through the security lines, clearly not well. Without assistance, I would slump to the floor. Then again, maybe the LA airport security staffers have a higher tolerance for passengers looking the way I do. Maybe I look like a severely hungover celeb, minus the alcohol, the hangover, the sunglasses, the coolness, and that celebrity part. Once I'm on the airplane, I sleep during the entire late-night, cross-country flight. I remember almost nothing about it, although I'm told that my children, their brows furrowed, keep peeking over the seat to check that I am still breathing and that I do not require emergency medical attention.

We get home on a Friday evening and I spend all of Saturday lying on the sofa in our cheery, orange-colored sunroom. I look washed out and exhausted even though I've just been on vacation. With my brother away on his own summer vacation at Cape Cod, it falls on Scott and the boys to drive my father home from the rehabilitation center as medical staffers there believe he's grown strong enough to go home. Luckily, Dad no longer needs to use a cane to get around, is eating well, and seems more alert. Scott texts and calls me throughout the day to both check up on me—he left me in Abbey's care—and to report on my father, saying he's encouraged by what he sees. A sure sign of hope: Dad asks Scott to drive the four of them to the famed White Hut in his hometown, where Dad is fond of the hot dogs smothered with the caramelized onions. Dad tries to persuade Casey to get onions on his burger but Casey, the picky eater who is swayed by nothing and no one, takes a pass on the onions.

"It made me nervous that he was so skinny," Jonah says later about my father, "but because he was so excited and energetic, I figured he was feeling better. He just wanted to assure us that he was okay. He was acting pretty confident."

By the time the three of them get home, I am asleep on the sofa. Scott gently helps me go upstairs to bed. My gait is unsteady. My head still feels fuzzy, like just-woke-up-after-taking-Nyquil-fuzzy.

The following morning, I wake up to that back-of-the-head pain, the dizziness, the weakness, the vomiting. After getting sick and then trying to return to my bed a few times, my energy is spent. Instead, I lie on the cold black tile of my bathroom floor to which my head feels magnetically drawn. I cannot lift it because when I do the pain I experience inside the back of my head is searing and I violently vomit. I am cemented in place as my legs go numb.

Scott comes in, doesn't like the sight of me on the floor, and tries to lift me up. I don't have the energy to fight him, but when my head comes off the floor, I vomit. He can't move me without me vomiting.

When I can no longer take the head pain, the whole-body weakness, the dizziness, and the vomiting—I have nothing left but acid—I beg Scott to call 9-1-1. This is now too big for us to handle on our own.

Here's what I remember from this point on:

I recall at least two EMTs entering the bathroom which is adjacent to my bedroom. (Scott and the kids remember three

EMTs entering the house.) One of them is behind me, lifting me up by holding me beneath my arms. When my head shifts into an upright position, my knees buckle, and I briefly faint.

The EMTs slide me onto a stretcher as I awaken and retch. One of the guys hands me a small plastic bag into which I can get sick, but very little is emerging from my mouth anymore. I am vaguely aware of being strapped in and carried down the stairs, out my front door, and past my three kids who are seeing their mother, for the third time in a week, weakened and unable to function. This time, I'm being carried away by strangers.

I remember the morning July sun, feeling a light breeze on my arms and feeling exposed in my driveway, in my sleeveless black cotton nightgown, lying on a stretcher, and sticking a plastic bag under my mouth every thirty seconds as nausea overcomes me. (Later, my neighbors send me a "Get Well" card telling me they saw me being loaded into an ambulance and were worried.)

The kids, uniformly, later tell me they were utterly confused and scared, particularly because Scott, who was busy packing up stuff and taking off in his car to follow the ambulance, hadn't told them much of anything about what was happening. Then again, Scott didn't really know what was happening.

According to the kids, Scott warned them before the EMTs arrived and asked them to take our dog Max and clear the way for them to get into the house. Abbey said the door to my bedroom remained closed—leaving her to wonder what was really going on—until the paramedics arrived. But the kids all heard the retching and the concerned tone of their father's voice.

"Dad tried to keep us in the kitchen and out of the way," Abbey said. "We were expecting Dad to go with you. We figured we were going with you."

But they do not accompany me in the ambulance, nor do

they join Scott in his car. They are left behind to fend for themselves for the day, to sit with their questions, their worry, their confusion, the nearly-thirteen-year-old and the two nearly-sixteen-year-olds.

"No one told me what was happening," said Casey, who was a rising eighth grader at the time. "I didn't know why you were sick so much that you had to go to the hospital. I just thought you had a pretty bad flu."

"We all kind of hung out together," Abbey added, saying they were unified by their mutual anger that their father had left them in the dark about what was going on.

Meanwhile, I am not at the local hospital very long before they transfer me to a Boston hospital for evaluation. The local emergency room physicians decide—given my statement that multiple lesions have been found in my brain and spine in a recent MRI—to pass me on to the hospital where Dr. Walker works. A different two-person ambulance crew drives me twenty-something miles into the city, my second ambulance ride of the day, to a hospital with so many underground hallways, twisty turns, and additions that I am never sure where I am in the building as my gurney is wheeled from floor to floor.

The first place I remember is being in the Emergency Room where I am evaluated by an ER neurologist. I've finally stopped retching but protectively cling to the small blue plastic bag wrapped around a plastic ring that I was given at the first hospital. I tell the ER neurologist guy what happened, working backwards chronologically, from the past few hours, the trip home from California, what happened in LA.

For the first time, I say out loud, "I believe I have MS. My recent MRI showed several lesions including new, active ones. I'm supposed to see my neurologist in two days."

What the ER neurologist doesn't tell me outright is that he thinks I am having an MS attack. It's only by reading my medical records later that I learn he had indeed reached the same conclusion as I did. It's right there, in the first line of his notes: "45F [45-year-old female] with new diagnosis of MS ... [R]ecent imaging reportedly now showing multiple demyelinating lesions." He described me as "mildly uncomfortable appearing" and noted that my speech was "slow but fluent." His diagnosis: vertigo and MS.

At some point in the evening, I'm admitted to the hospital and wheeled into a two-patient room on the neurology floor. I am assigned the bed next to the window, while the bed closest to the door is occupied by the woman whose head is covered by sensors that are connected by wires to a machine that is monitoring her brain for seizures. That's why she's in the hospital. Seizures. She has a gigantic personality. Even confined to the hospital bed, this woman has an outsized presence. She's funny, talkative, and exceedingly friendly, way more friendly and into swapping stories than I'm feeling at the moment. Oh, and she tells me she's a medium, meaning she can read people's auras and concerns, and communicate with the otherworld. When a team of med students and residents makes the rounds, for example, she reaches her hand out to one of the interns, "It's okay. You don't need to be afraid, honey. Go ahead and do your exam." The intern cocks her head to the side quizzically. "I can sense your fear, read it. Don't worry," my roommate says.

Over on the other side of Room 1109, where I can gaze out at the view of other medical buildings in Boston, I face away from her. Once the medical entourage sent to evaluate her leaves our room, I succumb to a wave of self-pity and irrational fear.

Don't read me. Don't read my thoughts! I think, as hard as I can think, as loudly as I can inside my damaged brain. *Just in case* my roommate can actually "hear" my thoughts. It's ridiculous, I know. I don't believe in mediums, but, then again, I don't believe what's happening to me either.

〜

The general neurologist who takes over my case once I'm on the neurology floor eyes me in the same way Dr. Sabine did years ago, giving off a disbelieving vibe. An older gentleman with aggressively bushy eyebrows, Dr. Roberts asks me the garden variety questions neuro patients usually get asked: "Who's the president?" "What's today's date?" "Where are we right now?" He conducts a very cursory physical exam, assessing my eye movement, the strength in my hands, my legs. He's mild-mannered but very aloof.

Later, I read the medical notes which explain what Dr. Roberts, the attending neurologist, really thinks: "The symptoms from the recent morning do not sound like those of a new MS lesion." While he says I should have a lumbar puncture and a new MRI, he writes, "… [T]here is no new symptom that suggests an MS lesion."

To my knowledge, no one has contacted Dr. Walker, despite my repeated requests that someone reach out to him. (Dr. Walker tells me later he doesn't recall hearing from his general neuro colleagues during my in-patient treatment.) No one with a medical license has officially told me that I have MS yet, I can only say that I think, based on what Dr. Walker has said, that I'm having an MS attack. The only person who seemed to believe me was the ER neurologist.

⌒

I have a CT scan of my head and chest. The scans are clean. I have an echocardiogram. It is uneventful. My blood is drawn. My urine is cultured. Bits of me are carted away for analysis, for answers. I am still weak but I'm no longer suffering from shattering nausea. I can eat, but just a little bit. I take a selfie from my cell phone and send it to my kids to show them that I'm still alive, even though my eyes look puffy and squinty, and my smile looks fake. I pointedly do not post anything on social media, although I do exchange a small number of texts with people from my hospital bed.

Scott spends hours in the room with me each day, brings me the daily newspapers that are delivered to our house, nervously gnaws on his fingernails, and replies to business emails from his phone, explaining to his colleagues that he can't make meetings. He spreads the word about my hospitalization to a handful of friends who, in turn, tell other friends. He calls Sean, who is vacationing at the Cape with his family and who arranges for a meal from a local restaurant to be delivered to the house for the kids to eat. My pal Gayle is in Washington, D.C. with her family and asks me if she should book a flight to Boston; I tell her, "No," that I'll likely be sprung from the hospital soon. My mother-in-law calls me, with a tearful and fearful edge to her voice, and tells me how much she's hoping things will turn out okay.

I only see one of the kids while I'm in the hospital. On the first full day I'm there, Jonah and Abbey have prearranged outings with friends that I don't want them to cancel. Later that evening, Casey accompanies Scott for a brief visit. The almost-thirteen-year-old tries valiantly to camouflage his worry and fear. He tries, but largely fails. It's not lost on me that the next day is this kid's birthday, for which Scott and I are utterly unprepared. The weekend we were going to use to get his gifts and ingredients for a cake, was consumed by my recovery, my father's release from rehab, and my hospitalization.

One of my friends whom Scott has texted, Sharon, visits me in the hospital in the latter end of the stay and brings me flowers. Our children have grown up together and we've seen one another through a lot of life events over the years. Her presence is a tremendous comfort, as she's one of those people with whom I can just be honest, be my vulnerable self, and not feel ashamed about my many faults. While she's there, a young med student, an intern I believe—someone with a warm smile and long brown hair—enters the room and tells me she's there to do a lumbar puncture, sometimes called a spinal tap. At the time of my hospitalization, some multiple sclerosis websites include lumbar punctures as one of the last-resort measures for diagnosing the disease. The Mayo Clinic's website describes the procedure as inserting a long needle entering the patient's lower back, in the lumbar area. "During the lumbar puncture," the website says, "a needle is inserted between two lumbar bones (vertebrae) to remove a sample of cerebrospinal fluid—the fluid that surrounds your brain and spinal cord to protect them from injury." Of the analysis of cerebrospinal fluid, the National Multiple Sclerosis Society says "by itself cannot confirm or rule out a diagnosis of MS. It must be part of the total clinical picture that takes into account the findings of the person's history and neurologic exam as well other diagnostic procedures."

This resident has the best bedside manner of anyone I've seen in the hospital thus far, with the exception of ER neurologist I met upon my arrival. She's utterly cheerful and personable. I do not feel at all anxious when she asks Sharon to step out of the room and asks me to hunch forward over the patient table as she exposes my back. "Ooh, you have a good back for this, a good back," she says reassuringly.

As the local anesthetic is administered, I silently hope the test will give me answers, answers I've been wanting since I was lying on a blanket in a Santa Monica park, since I was sitting in Dr. Sabine's office two years ago and he made me feel like a lunatic with a tenuous grip on reality. Then I abruptly stop thinking about the promise of getting answers about MS because a ghastly agony overloads my senses and commandeers my thoughts. Sharp pain travels up and down my spine.

No one said this test would be excruciating.

I hear the resident grumble under her breath, frustrated, while she works the needle. It feels as though thin threads of my spinal cord are being tugged, marionette strings trying to make me dance. I am gritting my teeth and digging my fingernails into the palms of my hands, but I cannot suppress the groans which involuntarily escape my mouth.

"Are you okay?" the young woman asks, her voice wavering.

"I just want you to finish it!" I snap. I normally don't snap at people, but this is horrifically painful.

She suggests I change positions. I lie down on my right side on the bed and draw my knees up to my chest so I'm comma-shaped, although I feel like an exclamation point of distress. She tries to administer the lumbar puncture again, but the fiery, yanking sensation is back

What is she doing? Is she grabbing nerve ending with Crate & Barrel salad tongs? I wonder.

I hear the resident behind me making sounds that concern me. This is clearly not going well. She says something about the test not working, blurts, "I'm sorry!" then tearfully runs out of the room. She had promised to fetch my friend Sharon from the family waiting room when the test was over, but she never does. I do not see this resident again.

Dr. Walker, who later tells me he doesn't use lumbar punctures to diagnose his patients with MS, says that as a physician, he's had the misfortune of conducting lumbar punctures that wound up failing. When he has done "unsuccessful" punctures in the past, he says, "I feel this stress rising, rising. The patient starts squirming more and more" and then he has had to call it off.

My discharge papers rather cryptically describe what happened with the lumbar puncture. "LP attempted by failed on 7/28/2014." It continues, "While in the hospital, lumbar puncture was attempted but unsuccessful due to pt's back anatomy."

But I thought I had a good back.

⤶

I have a urinary tract infection. The doctors discover this after they screen my urine. This positive test, the only positive test I had during my time in the hospital—the lumbar puncture yields an insignificant amount of cerebrospinal fluid—is just what Dr. Roberts, he of the bushy eyebrows, needs to close my case. In his discharge summary, Dr. Roberts wrote of the symptoms that sent me to the hospital that they were "resolved with intravenous fluid repletion and were attributed to a viral infection." "Discharge diagnosis: viral illness, UTI." My discharge papers did acknowledge that new lesions had been found in my brain recently, in particular, "an active enhancing lesion in the left cerebellar white matter." Several multiple sclerosis websites say that lesions in the cerebellum are associated with a host of symptoms including loss of balance, dizziness, vertigo, and nausea. A British patient website is even more specific, "Cerebellar lesions can produce nausea and/or vomiting. Sudden vomiting (without warning) after a positional change, without preceding nausea, is suggestive of a posterior fossa [in or near bottom of skull] lesion."

Less than an hour after being discharged, Scott drives me to Dr. Walker's satellite office in a Boston suburb. It's the first time I've been outdoors since my ambulance ride. I'm unsteady on my feet and shield my eyes from the sun. I have no idea where my sunglasses are.

"So, does she have MS?" Scott asks as we're still lowering ourselves into adjacent chairs in Dr. Walker's office.

"Well," Dr. Walker pauses, squints his eyes and knits his brow, "*ye-aaaah*." He might as well have replaced "yeah" with "duh." His tone sounds as if we should have already known this, like it was obvious to anyone who was paying attention.

Boom.

There it is.

I have multiple sclerosis. It *is* in my head, literally not metaphorically, not simply on an emotional basis. No hedging. No hesitation.

Dr. Walker conducts a physical exam but I'm kind of floating through it, over it, atop it, like I'm surfing on this new information. Waves, curling ferocious ones, swirl beneath me, drowning out everything else. He's testing my reflexes, my arm and leg strength, my vision, my dexterity. In my mind, I'm somewhere else entirely.

There is a discussion about medications, but everything is obscured by that "*ye-aaaah*" from Dr. Walker. Thick pamphlets, booklets really, are handed to me. I accept them but don't look at them, allowing them fall softly onto my lap. Long, complicated prescription brand names are bandied about: Tecfidera, Tysabri, Copaxone, Gilenya, Aubagio. Dr. Walker seems to favor Tecfidera, a new and powerful oral medication which has provided positive results to his patients. I really do not want to have to take injectable medication. That's one of the few things of which I'm certain.

I nod like I understand. I know nothing about any of these medications. I have trouble, initially, pronouncing their names. The pros and cons of the medicines that Dr. Walker explains fall out of my mind like grains of sand through a sieve. He tells me I need a blood test before I leave the office and that I should have another MRI as soon as I can schedule it at the hospital. I dutifully contribute more of my blood to the cause. "... [W]ith recent MRI data," Dr. Walker writes in a letter to my primary care physician on the day he sees me, "it is clear that she carried the diagnosis of [relapsing remitting multiple sclerosis]. It was unclear that she had any new neurological flare associated with recent [hospital] admission."

I stumble, literally, outside, back into my life, my new life as an MS patient. And it's Casey's thirteenth birthday. So, on top of feeling as though my ill-health marred the family's vacation, traumatized the kids with the ambulance ride and hospital stay, I am sick on Casey's birthday. Scott and I immediately go from Dr. Walker's office to one of Casey's favorite barbecue joints to pick up a large take-out order I place over the phone while en route. We get several pints of mac-and-cheese, tangy pulled chicken, pulled pork, sweet potato pudding with pecans and brown sugar on top, corn bread, and corn on the cob, a veritable spread on which the newly-minted teen could feast.

When we get home, we discover that the fixings for a "lava" cake Casey wants for his birthday are all set to be assembled, courtesy of my friend Gretchen, who will forever be called "the lady who saved Casey's thirteenth birthday." She didn't just provide the brownies, the vanilla ice cream, the whipped cream, and the hot fudge required to put together the cake (modeled after the dessert of the same name from The Rainforest Café), she bought birthday presents for us to give Casey. Scott and Gretchen had arranged for her to take all three of the kids for the day, something Scott forgets to tell the kids in advance. Casey was occupied by hanging out with Gretchen's younger son Colin, had lunch and played basketball with friends at a nearby court. Meanwhile, Gretchen took her older son Dustin and her daughter Grace, along with Abbey and Jonah to buy birthday presents for Casey so Scott and I will have something to give him when I get home from the hospital. She feeds them, keeps them busy, buys the birthday gifts, AND prepares the ingredients for his birthday cake. Her halo gleams especially brightly on this particular day.

As our family of five gathers around our kitchen table and digs into the barbecue, Casey tells us all about the awesome day he had with his friends. His mouth full of mac-and-cheese, Casey declares, "This is the best birthday ever!"

⌒

I'm trapped inside a face cage again, this time, at an MRI facility at the Boston hospital where Dr. Walker works. During the pre-procedure questioning the tech conducts with patients, I now have a clear answer for why this test was ordered: I have MS. I have to get used to saying this. It is no longer a question. It is a fact. This fact means that the long list of common and less common MS symptoms I read on the National Multiple Sclerosis Society's website could become my reality. Any of it or all of it. I cannot absorb the enormity of this. I can no longer picture my future. It is a vast void, splashed with white primer.

A little more than two weeks after my official diagnosis, I'm back in Dr. Walker's MS unit in the hospital. In the days since I've been released from the hospital, I have continued to experience intermittent lightheadedness to the point where I walk kind of funny, like I'm drunk. I have headaches, numbness in parts of my body, and a new, prickly feeling in the palms of my hands as well as my big toes. Since mid-June, when I had the MRI whose results Dr. Walker gave me over the phone when I was in California, I learn that two additional lesions have developed, a 6 x 4 mm lesion in the left midbrain and a 5 mm lesion in the right middle cerebellar peduncle, according to my lab reports. The lesion on the cerebellum is inflamed. Dr. Walker tells me I'm having, and probably have been having, what's called a multiple sclerosis flare-up, which also goes by a variety of other names including an MS attack, exacerbation, or relapse. Attacks can last for days or weeks. During an attack, the symptoms blossom in intensity. "An exacerbation of MS ... causes new symptoms or the worsening of old symptoms," the National Multiple Sclerosis Society website says. "It can be very mild, or severe enough to interfere with a person's ability to function at home and at work. ... To be a true exacerbation, the attack must be at least twenty-four hours and be separated from the previous attack by at least thirty days. Most exacerbations last from a few days to several weeks or even months."

To tamp down the inflammation and decrease the severity of this current attack, which has likely been going on since the California trip, Dr. Walker prescribes three days of steroid

IV infusions. Each infusion will take about an hour and the first one will occur right after I leave his office, he tells me. The steroids are a powerful weapon, Dr. Walker says, one that should be used sparingly, lest it cause other potentially damaging, long-term side effects such as diabetes, osteoporosis, arthritis, and cataracts. But with the speed at which the lesions are multiplying, he wants to act quickly. And, after so much uncertainty, things seem to be moving swiftly now that my diagnosis has been confirmed, now that we know what I'm facing. Not a case of nerves. Not a UTI.

Multiple. Sclerosis. Part of me wants to go back to the physicians who made me question myself, who suggested I wasn't *really* experiencing what I was reporting, and shove my new MRI scans in their smug faces. "It's multiple sclerosis, you ass holes," I fantasize about shouting.

But I have more important things to think about, like starting medicine to attempt to arrest the progression of the disease, which has been moving quickly since June. Having finally read through the literature Dr. Walker gave me about not only MS but the different disease-modifying medications that are available, I am now comfortable with his recommendation: a relatively new oral medication called Tecifidera (TECK-fid-dare-a), otherwise known as dimethyl fumarate. I'll take it twice daily. It's supposed to prevent new brain and spinal lesions from forming, to extend the time between MS exacerbations, and to reduce the intensity of the symptoms during flare-ups.

Oral MS treatments have only been around for a couple of years. Prior to that, MS patients had to inject medicine daily with hypodermic needles, or regularly received chemotherapy or steroids to treat the disease. There were no treatments before the early 1990s when patients just suffered. On paper, Tecfidera seems to be the best option for me but I will have to see how my body reacts to the aqua-colored capsules. The side effects, as with most medicines—you've seen those unnerving drug ads on TV with the super-fast-talking warnings—are daunting. One biggie with this medicine is gastrointestinal problems including: nausea, vomiting, diarrhea, and stomach pain. My stomach is already an unstable mess as my tendency to worry about everything plays out squarely in my gut. Throwing a strong medicine into the mix, well, that gives me even more to worry about, if you don't count the incurable autoimmune disease that could render me deaf, blind, speechless, and in a wheelchair as reasons to worry.

Some patients tolerate Tecfidera well; others are debilitated by it. I have no idea which one I'll be. Dr. Walker prescribes additional medicine to help with nausea and another for abdominal cramping just in case that's what happens once I pop those pills. Oh, and here's another fun fact from the official Tecfidera website, it "may cause serious side effects including allergic reactions, PML, which is a rare brain infection that usually leads to death or severe disability, and decreases in your white blood cell count." I add that to the list of things about which I can fret.

～

My fingertips feel abnormally heavy and my eyes feel as though they're taking a beat too long to adjust when I shift my gaze from one thing to another, like from the book I'm reading to the nurse who's walking into the room at the end of my three-day course of IV steroids. I have spotty dizziness. The soles of my feet are numb as are the palms of my hands. When I walk, I suspect that I look inebriated because I'm so unsteady on my feet. The insomnia the nurses said I might experience as a result of the steroids hits me on the night after the final infusion. I get up at three in the morning and watch bad TV even though I crave the shuteye.

I try to keep spirits up by cracking wise about this situation, but no one seems to find amusing my jokes about becoming all Hulk-like because of the steroids, about my muscles suddenly bulging and busting through my clothing like it is mere tissue paper. The jokes are likely lame, given that they're being delivered by a pale-faced, weak-looking, middle-aged woman who is stumbling around, but this is the only way I can think of to try to make this seem okay. Prompting laughter, even if it's just my own, feels like the only thing I can control right now.

AFTER

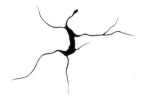

CHAPTER NINE
The Little Aqua Blue Pill

It takes me by surprise, this being stripped of control over my body business. Maybe it shouldn't, given my earlier struggles with infertility, but having now had three children, those visceral fears faded into the background. This MS diagnosis is an unwelcomed reminder of the arrogant fallacy in which I'd been indulging, that one can determine what will happen in one's future. We never really have control. We just don't like to admit our powerlessness as we vainly make our plans in our eighteen-month calendars, make projections for our retirement savings, craft our overconfident five-year plans for people and organizations ... plans which, at this moment in my life, seem only as powerful as the thin pieces of paper upon which they're printed. Try as we might—consuming mass amounts of kale and exercising every day, avoiding cigarettes and alcohol and fatty foods—cannot completely protect us from getting sick. Sure, they can sweeten our odds of being healthy, but we can't do anything about whether we are predisposed to go bald, to get wrinkles, to develop bad backs, or develop cancer. As we grow older and witness friends and family cope with illnesses and physical ailments that seem to crop up out of nowhere, we realize some individuals are simply better equipped than others at allowing these turns of fate to roll off their shoulders, to accept our innate helplessness about the destinies of our bodies.

In my case, I'm not currently doing so well with the unpredictable, incurable disease that has taken the picture I had created in my mind of my potential future and vaporized it. Over a period of months in 2014, I go from being a healthy—albeit anxious—woman in her mid-forties, to being forever a "patient," someone with a chronic, capricious, and frequently degenerative illness that is listed as a disability on job applications. During that same period, my mother died, my father's health declined, and my teaching contract was not renewed because, as they said, I didn't possess the right degree. As I obsess about the change the official diagnosis is making to my self-image and my daily life, I acknowledge that, in many ways, I am wildly blessed by several important things. I'm blessed that I have three healthy children, a caring spouse, and kind friends. But, in light of my recent diagnosis, I'm keenly aware of two other blessings: our family's health insurance policy, obtained through Scott's work, and the federal Affordable Care Act, which made it illegal to deny health insurance coverage for anyone due to a "pre-existing condition." Should Scott ever change (or lose) his job, I can still get health insurance coverage without being denied or charged exorbitant fees that could bankrupt my family simply because of my MS diagnosis. Without health insurance, the prescription for the aqua blue Tecfidera pills that are supposed to help keep my MS from quickly worsening, my family would have to shell out $60,000 per year, roughly $82 per pill, and I take two pills per day. (By 2017, the annual cost of this medication rises to the dunning price of $83,000 per year as Congress and the president make repeated attempts to repeal large swaths of the Affordable Care Act but have yet to do so. By 2019, the market rate for Tecfidera is nearly $100,000 a year.)

The price tag for my MS medicine, Tecfidera, chills me. I pray that my health insurance policy will continue to cover the lion's share of the cost, as well as help pay for the expensive MRIs I will need to assess how my disease is progressing and whether the medicine is working. If we were to lose our health insurance—or if I was to lose the legal protection of the law which makes it illegal to discriminate against me when it comes to health insurance—my family could not pay for this medicine and this treatment for the rest of my life. Multiple sclerosis is chronic and I will need to take this disease-modifying medication until it stops working, at which case, I'll have to move on to another treatment. I will be getting "treatment," to ward away the development of new lesions and to try to keep MS attacks at bay, until a cure is found. Without it, the rest of my life would likely be comprised of bits of time between incidents like what happened at the Hollywood Bowl and the one that sent me to the hospital, as I slowly get sicker. Without the treatment, I risk permanent damage to my nerves and I would potentially compromise my ability to get around, to work. To avoid those things, or at least to try, I need tens of thousands of dollars of prescription drugs and treatment every year. It's expensive to be an MS patient. So, every time I hear national politicians threaten to remove the legal protections for those people who have pre-existing conditions or to do away with prescription drug coverage, I panic inside, worrying that, in the future, my ill health will not just break my heart, but will bankrupt my family.

The monumental blessings of health insurance aside—without it, this would be an entirely different tale—starting this MS medicine, Tecfidera, means more than just creating a new daily routine I *absolutely* need to remember. In the first few weeks of taking Tecfidera, I will be on edge, uncertain as to what side effects, if any, I will experience.

Will I be chained to the house, debilitated by abdominal cramping, diarrhea or vomiting? Will I succumb to that fatal brain infection I read about online?

In online forums, some MS patients who have used this medication report that the drug is akin to carpet-bombing their immune systems, compromising them to the point where immunity to other diseases is almost non-existent. Since the medicine attempts to stop patients' broken immune systems from attacking their brain and spinal cord, it simultaneously suppresses the functioning parts of patients' immune systems. A number of patients report the medicine makes them so sick that they switched to a different drug treatment. Given the ambiguity about how I am going to react to this relatively new medication, I opt to stop seeking a new teaching position. For now.

In the meantime, the question of whether I'll be well enough, clear-headed enough to plunge, full-throttle into writing the book about the middle school jazz band in mourning looms large. I don't know what to say to people when they ask whether I've made any progress on it because I'm not broadcasting the diagnosis on a wide basis right now. To the outside world, I fear I come off as a pampered sloth because I'm not employed, haven't produced the book about the jazz band yet, and am spending a lot of time at home. I worry about what people think, especially when I tell them I won't be teaching in the fall. But I'm more concerned with what I think about myself.

Without my teaching, without my writing, what am I?

In the heat of August 2014—as I continue to experience fatigue, lightheadedness, and nausea while I walk around my air-conditioned house—inside I am boiling in self-pity. I'm angry that I'm not going to be stepping in front of a classroom in the fall, angry that my mother is dead, that my father is paralyzed by grief. I'm angry that my own combination of grief and illness has pushed my writing, my working on the book, onto the backburner, angry that I can't picture anything beyond the next day, angry that I have this meaty question mark dangling over me: *What can I control here?*

I survey the year's wreckage, sift through the pieces of my former life, and examine events that still do not seem real to me. Intellectually, I do not want to wallow in self-indulgent despondency, as justifiable as it may seem to me while I stare blankly out the window of our orange sunroom into the moist summer air. However, my emotions are running amok.

I can write. I am a writer, I tell myself. *Even if I get tired, even if I encounter vision problems, I can still write, can't I?*

The reason I was given for not getting reappointed to my two-year, temporary teaching position was my lack of a terminal degree in my field. Despite years of writing, reporting, and teaching experience at the collegiate level, it came down to having the "right" piece of paper. This is something with which I become preoccupied in the waning days of the summer of 2014, when I am not thinking about my health. This fixation makes it easier for me to decide what I will do now that I'm so uncertain as to in what shape my health will be for the very near future. To stave off a growing sense of despair, I hastily make a decision: in addition to finishing the book about the band—to which I have given the working title, *Mr. Clark's Big Band*—I need a little something else to keep me going and moving forward.

I have to move forward. I cannot stay here, stuck in this failure, in this illness, in this grief.

Without doing a whole lot of research, without making one of my pros-and-cons lists, I impulsively apply to an online MFA writing program in creative nonfiction. I decide that the jazz band book will be my thesis. Through a professional connection and sheer serendipity, within two weeks of this epiphany in the sunroom, I enroll in an online MFA creative nonfiction program where students will have rigorous deadlines, will be expected to participate in mandatory bulletin boards for dialogue, critiques, and observations, and must join the occasional online conference calls and video chats. I do not have to show up to classes in person. I can write from wherever I am. This works perfectly for me in this peculiar moment in my life; if I suffer debilitating side effects from my new medicine, I can write from bed and no one will be the wiser. Worst case scenario: if I cannot concentrate and become too sick, I will take a medical leave of absence. I will work on *Mr. Clark's Band Book* steadily through the program and receive important feedback along the way. Although MS has stolen my vision of the future from me, I want to fight back.

This could work, I think optimistically.

A former newspaper colleague of mine, an author who blurbed my novel a few years ago, helped design the program at this western Massachusetts university and serves as its writer-in-residence. When I inquire about the program, her enthusiasm bursts through our email correspondence like a confetti bomb. Via email, she introduces me to the program director and, suddenly, I'm an MFA student.

Provided that MS doesn't take away my cognitive abilities, I can still be a writer, I tell myself, crossing my fingers so I don't jinx myself. *I can get this band book done AND get that piece of paper, that terminal degree.*

While I cling to my identity as a writer like a drowning woman to a life raft, I haven't accepted that I'm also the writer who takes two pricey pills a day with a tablespoon of peanut butter in the morning and evening (the peanut butter protects my stomach lining from the potentially corrosive effects of the new drug). I haven't yet familiarized myself with phrases like the "MS hug," a cloying nickname for an uncomfortable tightening around a patient's abdomen and back. In real life, the MS hug feels like someone is trying to fasten a too-tight corset around me to the point where it's hard to breathe ... all because some protective lining of nerves in my brain is damaged, not because I've strained anything. There's nothing adorable about it. I also haven't come to terms with the many aspects of the way I live my life must now change.

If I had not been in denial about the immediate necessity to change the way I move through and interact with the world, I would have realized that attending a Boston Red Sox game on an extremely hot and muggy early September night and parking a fifteen-minute walk from Fenway Park is a bad idea because, for some MS patients, heat and humidity can temporarily aggravate symptoms and make you feel like you're having an MS attack. Remember what happened in Santa Monica? How I was lying in the Palisades Park unable to lift my head as I retched? That's what now happens to me when I'm in weather like that, only I'm not allowing rational thoughts to permeate my stubbornness, my insistence that I cling to my old life and my old, pre-multiple sclerosis days. I want to be the same baseball fan who has watched Sox games in all kinds of weather—from damp and freezing April evenings, to scorching late August afternoons. I do not want to be someone who's sick, so I suppress the details of my new reality as Scott and I park at the Prudential Center, like we have many times before going to Fenway. This is my first real outing since my two-day hospitalization, and I am excited. I long to feel "normal," just another member of Red Sox Nation taking in a game. But I am post-diagnosis Meredith, not healthy Meredith, a fact with which I will be forced to acknowledge sooner rather than later.

One of my favorite views in the world is the one you get when you walk up the ramp which takes you from inside the concrete Fenway Park concourse to the ballfield. When you lay your eyes on the majestic, manicured grass, it seems to rise toward the heavens in front of you. The anticipation of that first glimpse—no matter how many times I've been to Fenway—always feeds my excitement as I head to the park. It brings me back to the days when I was a young fan in a Dorothy Hamill haircut, proudly sporting my navy 1970s Red Sox jacket with the red piping down the sleeves and a bread plate-sized button bearing the face of star right fielder Dwight Evans pinned on the front. That little kid enthusiasm still lives within me.

But walking down Boylston Street on this September evening, in this new period of my life, I'm not thinking about Fenway's verdant grass because the muscles in my usually sturdy legs feel as though they've been infused with jelly. I am sweating even though we're not walking that fast. Tiny white spots are beginning to crowd my peripheral vision, like my own private showing of shooting stars that linger and flicker, nothing upon which I can make a wish. If I had been a cartoon character, my head would have floated upward, tethered by a thin, sinuous cord of damaged nerves. I would look down on myself from above and watch as my gait becomes almost comically unsteady, like I am awkwardly sloshing forward through knee-high water. But Boylston Street is not flooded. That ridiculously-named MS hug starts to squeeze my abdomen and my breathing becomes labored. I stop walking, bend at the waist, and brace my arms against my knees. Scott—who doesn't understand what's happening, because I haven't told him that my body feels as though it's being rapidly short-circuited—offers to buy me a bottle of water from one of the street vendors who are positioned around the route to the ballpark, sitting atop beat-up coolers piled high with ice. Some noisy pedi-cabs, clanging their tinkling bells, pass by.

"You want to get one?" Scott asks, pointing to a pedi-cab. He's not very good at masking his concern. Given the events of the past several weeks, his concern is not that surprising. "If you don't feel well, we can get one." He's in problem-solving mode, hero-mode. And I'm having none of it. Hopping into a pedi-cab feels like an admission of failure, like a modified version of an ambulance ride to take me to Fenway because I can't get there of my own volition like I always have before. I stubbornly refuse to give in to my body's warning signs, even though reason is telling me I should take a break, that missing the beginning of the game isn't a big deal, that getting a ride isn't a sign of weakness, that fighting those corporeal warning signs is a fruitless waste of precious energy. I am not being reasonable. I come from obstinate stock. I shake off Scott's offer as I remain hunched over and quiet. We are nearly equidistant from the Prudential Center parking garage and Fenway

Park, stuck in between my former life and my new one. My reluctance to move forward into uncertainty is rooting me in place, paralyzing me.

When I feel strong enough to start walking again, we do so at the pace of someone in dire need of knee replacement surgery. I feel silly to be walking so slowly and so inelegantly when, to the rest of the world, it doesn't look like there's anything physically wrong with me. Looking at me, you wouldn't know that my immune system is at war with the nerves in my brain and spinal cord, that it is trying to destroy the channels of communication between them. My damage is invisible.

Later, while leafing through my MRI reports, I read that one of the lesions in the middle of my brain has a "dark hole." This stops me.

I have a dark hole in my brain. Kind of amusing, in a twisted sort of way. *Maybe I can blame my dark thoughts, my tendency to imagine the worst has happened when someone is late getting home, or my affection for pitch-black humor on this dark hole in my midbrain.* A medical web page I found later used the phrase "dark hole" synonymously with "black hole," and explained "black holes reflect irreversible demyelination and axonal [nerve] loss."

Dr. Walker later apologizes that this "very unfortunate term" is included in the radiology report. This kind of language, he says, unnecessarily frightens patients even though these dark areas most often indicate permanent nerve damage. But instead of using "black holes" or "dark holes," Dr. Walker says he uses "T1-hypointensity" because "that's less scary. ... Why say something that you don't need to say?"

That dark hole, along with the other lesions that are currently inflamed and not yet being treated by MS drugs, have changed me in ways I cannot see but can feel as I stand there on a steamy city sidewalk on an early autumn evening, being forced to face the truth.

We eventually make it to the ballpark on foot while moving at an absurdly slow pace. I don't inform Scott that I feel as why did you hide it?

though I'm going to faint or that my legs are about to give out. I am already tired of being the sick one for which he has to care, and we're only a month into this rest-of-my-life MS journey. I just want to get to our seats—which are great, by the way, on the third baseline—and have a cool drink. I post a photo of the two of us on Facebook, both smiling, me glistening with perspiration, glasses sitting in front of tired eyes, the beauty of Fenway illuminated by powerful lights behind us. The photo is a lie of some degree, like most of my social media posts in the weeks after my multiple sclerosis diagnosis, falsely projecting happiness and health. While I do enjoy the exciting game—it goes ten innings and the Sox beat the Blue Jays 9-8— I spend most of the time trying to regain my composure and equilibrium, impatiently waiting for those flashing spots in my eyes to fade, for my nausea to subside, my light-headedness to abate. On the inside, I am a mess.

Over the course of the three-plus-hour ballgame, my head eventually clears. I no longer feel dizzy or like I'm going to collapse. That's the good news. The bad news is that I discover a new symptom while sitting in the seats: a jolt of prickly electricity that zaps up and down my spine when I bend my neck and tilt my head forward. While picking up my purse from the ground in front of my seat, my neck and back feel momentarily electrified, not an unpleasant sensation, just, well, shocking, like pins and needles after a limb has fallen asleep. At home later, I look up the new symptom. It has a name. Lhermitte's Sign.

⁓

There's burning in the back of my head, specifically, on the right side. It's the same location that throbbed when I was hospitalized in July. I add this now-frequent symptom in a notebook where I'm keeping track of the growing constellation of symptoms upon which MS has given me: intermittent dizziness, head pain, nausea, overwhelming fatigue, leg weakness, spots in my vision, the MS hug, and Lhermitte's Sign.

I try to push the list of horribles out of my mind as I return to yoga classes in the fall of 2014 at a local studio, after a year-long hiatus from the practice. My pal Gretchen, the one who saved my son Casey's birthday, coaxes me back to my yoga mat. She has been very concerned about my condition and really wants to do something to help. Bringing me to yoga is something she can do. I don't mention that I'm worried about my symptoms, particularly the dizziness part, hindering my yoga practice. The last thing I want is to be in the tree position, lose my balance, keel over, and accidentally take out several classmates along with me. I do not want to get into the pigeon pose, have my legs go numb, and require people to pull me up off the floor. I am still frequently replaying in my head the scene in my bathroom when the EMTs lifted me up and I fainted. I am apprehensive about my ability to exercise in public without inadvertently becoming a humiliating spectacle. But Gretchen is persuasive. I dig my underused light green yoga mat from beneath the junk clogging up the shelves in the garage and put on my game face.

Upon entering the studio, I quietly inform the instructor I have recently been diagnosed with MS and may have some balance issues. (To be honest, balance has never been my strong suit even before MS. As a mediocre child gymnast, the balance beam was my worst event.) The instructor nods but I cannot tell if she understands. I will come to realize, as I slowly tell people about having MS, this is a typical reaction, this affirmative head-nodding. Most people do not seem to fully understand what it means to have MS. Most folks hear the name and envision wheelchairs, nursing homes, even death. I know that permanent disability is what my father thinks; the first words out of his mouth during every weekly phone call are, "How *are* you?" delivered with a sense of alarm rather than out of mundane, polite curiosity. (Years later, I will call him after returning home from an overseas trip. Having incorrectly written down wrong return date, he is panicked about why I haven't called him. "I thought you were in the hospital!" he will say urgently over the phone. To him, no matter what I tell him about the disease, I will always be on the precipice of hospitalization or en route to a wheelchair.)

I flatten my yoga mat on the cold floor. I keep telling myself that exercise is good for everybody, especially those with MS, or so I'd recently read in the packets of info that arrived in the mail from the National Multiple Sclerosis Society. However, I'm apprehensive about how this is going to play out, worried I'll be embarrassed. That I will fail. That everyone will see me fail, see me vulnerable. Despite my initial doubts, the first class is uneventful. Nobody, including me, was taken out on a stretcher, nor did anybody faint and take out a line of others who were trying to balance in dancer's pose. My body remembers the stretches, the poses, the breathing. I continue attending classes, once a week for several weeks in a row, even as the electric jolt I experience in my spine when I put my head down zaps me repeatedly during every session. When I get home from the yoga studio in the early evening, I experience bone-deep exhaustion. My thighs tingle for hours afterward, like they're heavy with buzzing bees. Still, I go to yoga because that's what everyone says I'm supposed to do. The exercise will help, I'm told repeatedly. I need to keep moving forward.

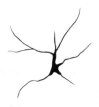

CHAPTER TEN

Fever Fatale

Newcomb Hollow Beach isn't our "regular" Cape Cod beach that we visit when we go to Wellfleet. Dad has always been very big on "regular," on finding something he likes—a beach, a restaurant—and sticking with it for as long as possible. Routines and reliability offer him tremendous comfort. But the ceremonial laying to rest of the remainder of Mom's ashes in the Atlantic Ocean will not take place at our "regular" beach, LeCount Hollow Beach, the Wellfleet beach where my father frolicked when he was a child in the 1950s, where Sean and I played in the 1970s, where my kids and nephews played in the late 1990s-early 2000s. On this brilliant October afternoon in 2014, when the sky is unnervingly blue, we do not put Mom's ashes to rest at the beach of my family's collective childhoods, despite Dad's fondness for the familiar.

With his bad knees, Dad says he can no longer scale LeCount Hollow's cliff-like dunes, can no longer set foot on the beach where, many years ago, my bikini-clad, chain-smoking mother used to slather herself with baby oil as she drank cans of beer in brazen violation of the no-booze rule on the Cape Cod National Seashore beaches, almost daring the eagle-eyed lifeguards to even *try* to confiscate the beer from her. She wasn't the type who went to the beach and devoured books like Dad, Sean, and me. Reading wasn't her thing, unless you counted magazines, especially cooking and fashion periodicals from which she'd rip pages and ambitiously circle items, recipes, or outfits, writing in her artistic cursive, "Need to try this!" She collected pages aspirationally torn from magazines with tips on how to make life more enjoyable, more beautiful. Mom also wasn't apt to join Sean, Dad, or me when we went swimming and body surfed in the flesh-numbingly cold Atlantic Ocean. There was no sand wedged beneath her painted fingernails from making sandcastles on the edge of the surf. When she went to the beach, Mom preferred to slip her oversized, Jackie Kennedy black sunglasses over her dark eyes, sip her beer, and cook her olive-toned skin to a sizzling deep brown, which looked amazing when she wore summer white, while listening to pop music on the portable radio. I could never be as cool, as confident as Mom in her bikini, in her tan, in her mani-pedi, not caring she was breaking the beach rules. Never.

Many decades removed from the days of Mom suntanning her baby oiled skin, Dad now has difficulty walking. Although LeCount Hollow has a nostalgic draw on Dad's memories, he asks Sean and me to select another Wellfleet beach at which we will deposit that Styrofoam-like water urn that Scott and I have stowed away in our garage since the day the other half of her ashes was interred in the cemetery. Dad really wants part of Mom to rest in Wellfleet because he is choosing to pluck happy, sun-splashed memories from his life with her from the family story and focus on them.

Even though it's the site of cherished childhood moments, Wellfleet is, to me, also a place that's inseparable from the vivid recollections I have of my mother's first battle with cancer—the one she won—where, after intense chemotherapy, her hair began falling out in clumps while we were on vacation. During the summer of 2000, Mom arrived at the Cape having already had the energy drained from her body by a vampire disguised as medical treatment. Her normally dark skin had gone pale with sickness, her fierce eyes hooded by fatigue and worry. One afternoon that July, my toddler twins napped inside the rented Wellfleet cottage—the one where you could see a sliver of the ocean at LeCount Hollow Beach if you stood on your toes at the back end of the wrap-around deck—as I watched my mother pull at her dark hair which was being blown away from her forehead by an ocean breeze. She looked slightly stunned as strands of hair easily released from her scalp while she ran her fingers through her bob hairstyle. Upon seeing the hair between her fingers, my father got upset and went inside.

Wellfleet's LeCount Hollow Beach also happens to be the site of Sean's near-drowning, although that family tale seems to nag away at my heart alone, as the person on whom blame for the entire incident was pinned. All these years later, that afternoon remains crystal clear to me and I still feel badly about it.

I'm guessing, however, that Dad prefers to remember the bold, tanned, beer-drinking version of his wife and that he has carefully expunged memories from his mind of that summer when Mom was ill. (One can only imagine the summertime memories my teenagers made while watching *their* mother fall ill in Los Angeles.) Maybe Dad wants to keep half of her close to home in that rural cemetery, and half of her floating in a never-ending, baby oil-scented, Cape Cod beach day. That's what I surmise anyway. I do not ask him why he decides to have this done because I cannot seem to gather the courage to pose the question. There hasn't ever seemed to be a good time to discuss it with him even though we speak regularly on the telephone. I don't know if I want to even ask because I'm not sure what the answer will be. And after a horrific summer where Dad, my nephew Sam, and I have all been hospitalized, I honestly do not have the emotional vigor to press for a reason why.

The beach Sean and I eventually select, Newcomb Hollow Beach, part of the Cape Cod National Seashore, is an eight-minute car ride down Ocean View Drive from LeCount Hollow.

Based on our internet research, it seems like it will be a good spot. Neither of us has had time to personally check out the beach in advance so we are relying on images we found online. We figure Dad can get down to the water since the dunes are not as steep as the ones at LeCount's. Considering that there are severe slopes at all of Wellfleet's National Seashore beaches, this is our best option. However, when we arrive in person on that warm October day, Dad takes one look at the sandy, descending path and informs us he will not attempt to walk the gentle decline to the water's edge. He is sixty-seven years old and has a host of physical ailments that have continued to plague him since he was released from the rehab center in July following his hospitalization, not counting the knees.

Five months after Mom's death, we are gathering to conduct one last ceremony to place her remains into the thunderous surf, the surf at which she used to gaze from behind her big sunglasses. The autumn weather is rather mild, mild enough for Sean, me, and our young families to doff our shoes, roll up our pant legs, and dip our feet into the salty water, not yet chilled by the frigid New England winter to come. Fortunately, Dad, clutching the weathered, wooden fence at the edge of the beach parking lot, is not standing sentry alone atop the dunes. He has his brother and one of his childhood friends with him to serve as solemn witnesses.

Sean and I walk a few feet away from our spouses and children, as we prepare to launch the urn into the water. My responsibility during this informal ceremony is to pour wine into the waves in honor of the Wine Mother. Prior to Mom's radio stint which earned her that moniker, she spent years trying to teach Sean and me about wine, quizzing us about what we smelled when we swirled our glasses, about what, *exactly*, we tasted during our initial sip. While Mom would educate us about acidity and the impact of the type of wood used in a wine barrel has on the ultimate taste of the wine, Dad would ruthlessly make fun of her solemnity. For example, when Mom would ask us to describe the Cabernet Sauvignon she was serving during a roast beef dinner, Dad, content in his role as the resident crackup, would make a big show of swirling his wine in the glass (a vessel specifically designed for red wine), take an exaggerated sitcom-like sniff, gulp down a sip, and declare, "Tastes like tar," then burst into laughter. Mom's lips would form a tight, straight line across her face as she glared at him across the oval kitchen table. Sean, with his refined palate, learned to offer the right answers to her questions, or, better yet, had the extraordinary gift of easily redirecting the conversation when he didn't. Me? While I didn't make fun of her earnestness when she discussed her life's passion, I am the Wine Mother's disappointing daughter, the one who couldn't discern the notes of apricot or smell the hints of oak in the Chardonnay or select the "right" wine to order at a restaurant. (The fact that, years from now, MS erodes my ability to taste a great many things, including certain wines, is not without irony for me.)

Yet I am the one tasked with bringing the wine to this event.

With my father bellowing directives at us into the wind— *Cut a hole in the bottom of the urn!* and *Hurry up! The tide's coming in!*—I worry the intact urn will break into pieces before we get it into the water and far enough from shore. I envision images of an errant wave smashing the flimsy off-white contraption to bits just at the point where the wave breaks and having charred bits of Mom wash back up onto our bare feet, something that I believe would deeply annoy her if she had the capacity to speak in anything other than our memories.

I brought an unimpressive varietal I bought at a local wine store for $15 and poured it into a one-liter plastic bottle that once contained lime-flavored seltzer water, which made for a distinctly less dramatic impression than uncorking a fresh bottle in the face of the waves would have done. Cognizant of the rules prohibiting alcohol on the beach, I wanted to camouflage the booze in case any officials, police, or National Park employees, happen to see us. Unlike Mom, I am always striving to be the rule-following, good girl and desperately do not want to get called out by law enforcement, particularly in front of my teenage children and my young nephews. So, I choose to hide the wine in a plastic bottle.

Coward, I imagine Mom muttering under her breath, as I meekly unscrew the seltzer bottle filled with that non-descript wine, and pour it into the water, instead of dramatically releasing a fabulous Cabernet with great relish. I wish that I had it in me to be brave like her and flout the rules, just like I wish I had it in me to speak at her funeral instead of doing what I did, silently stewing in a mélange of discomfort because I couldn't effectively put my feelings into cogent sentences at the time. Alas, words and flourish fail me at this moment too. As I am pouring out the wine, Sean hurls the urn into the sea from the shore of a beach that isn't our regular Cape Cod beach. I fret about the urn breaking prematurely, about getting caught with the wine at the beach, about my frail father clutching the split-rail fence at the top of the dune, about anything other than what is actually transpiring, the final act of putting her remains to rest.

The urn, as it turns out, doesn't immediately break when it lands in the water. At least we don't see it break. But we know that it eventually did, and Mom is now at rest in the sea.

〜

A fever could be life-threatening.

That line from an old episode of *The West Wing* prompts me to immediately Google whether, in fact, a fever is fatal to someone with relapsing remitting multiple sclerosis. Fresh from learning I have MS, this suggestion plunges me into a panic. A search of "fever and multiple sclerosis" in the fall of 2014 yields over 590,000 results. The first result comes from a website called Healthline, reporting on a study which discovered that patients who have low-grade fevers suffer more from chronic fatigue than others. The next result is an article saying many MS patients experience an exacerbation of symptoms when they're overheated, whether from the weather or fevers.

"In the old days, a hot-bath test was one of the ways doctors diagnosed MS," the Everyday Health website quotes a physician as saying. "MS symptoms, especially tingling, are usually worse in the summer because of the heat. Getting into air conditioning or taking a cool shower usually helps reduce heat symptoms."

But what about this life-threatening business? I mutter as I sit at my desk, freaking out over whether what I heard on the Emmy-winning Aaron Sorkin TV classic is indeed true. *Can a fever prove fatal as the fictional first lady says in the drama about a president who has relapsing remitting MS?* Would I, someone with the same unpredictable and incurable ailment, have to start wearing a mask in public to avoid getting sick? Cover myself in Purell? Keep a ten-foot protective perimeter from the walking petri dishes known as my grade school-aged nephews?

As I scan web page after web page and find nothing about a fever being a potentially fatal complication for people like me, I tentatively began to unclench my muscles. Just a wee bit. But I'm not satisfied with what I've found. I keep digging. I input "fever and multiple sclerosis and west wing" in the search box. The first result is "MS Goes 'West'" on a website called Mult-sclerosis.org. The piece explores whether NBC's *The West Wing*'s President Jed Bartlet character accurately represents the experiences of MS patients. While the article notes that the National Multiple Sclerosis Society bestowed an award on the program for raising awareness about the autoimmune disorder which attacks the central nervous system and, as of 2019 afflicts one million Americans a year, it only briefly mentions the fever issue which became a major plot point after President Bartlet (Martin Sheen), who is suffering an MS flare-up and passes out in the Oval Office. His wife Abbey, a physician, tearfully admits to a staffer that it isn't the flu that is making him ill.

"I see you trying to cover the panic," the chief of staff tells the *West Wing* first lady, imploring her to reveal what is really going on.

"He has multiple sclerosis Leo," Abbey Bartlet (Stockard Channing) says in a near-whisper. "... A fever could be life-threatening."

Abbey Bartlet's words echo inside my head, ping off my own damaged nerves. I am brimming with questions:

Will my own MS symptoms gradually worsen, or will they remain in an uncomfortable stasis as long as I continue taking my aqua-colored capsules twice a day? Will I eventually suffer cognitive anomalies, experience gait and walking problems, go blind, wind up in a wheelchair, suffer with chronic pain, or encounter speech, swallowing and incontinence problems that are among the rogue's gallery of woes which can befall MS patients?

Answers to my questions remain elusive.

The disease, which I've heard some describe as "quirky," does not manifest itself the same way in every patient. It's a matter of luck—or lack thereof—as to which nerves and areas of the brain and spinal cord become damaged by my immune system which is wreaking havoc on the protective layers of the nerves. If a lesion, only visible in MRIs, develops, say, in the optical area of the brain and interrupts the communication between my brain and my eyes, my vision may be temporary or permanently affected. If the area involved in memory gets targeted by the disease, I could start forgetting more than just signing my kids' permission slips for school trips or that it was my turn to make a homemade lasagna for a cross country team dinner. There's ADHD medicine to help if that happens, my neurologist tells me, but still, the thought of losing one's cognitive abilities is beyond disturbing.

In the aftermath of being newly diagnosed, I adopt certain new behaviors, like learning how to keep my body's temperature cool otherwise my symptoms will rush to the forefront and sabotage my day, potentially sending me to bed, the bathroom, the doctor ... or worse. After the experience at the muggy Red Sox game in September, I decide to skip many subsequent outdoor outings because it is too hot or muggy. I learn that I must be selective about which activities get my now-limited amounts of energy and oftentimes cancel events when I have no more energy to spare. In the prime of one's life, at the age of forty-five, the idea that my body's energy needs to be managed is a tough reality to swallow.

As I devour every new piece of information I can about the disease, I begin to take notice of pop culture and media references to MS. It is as if I am suddenly noticing things that have been there all along but previously ignored. It happens to everybody when anything out-of-the-ordinary or unexpected happens—you lose your job, you are trying to get pregnant and it doesn't happen right away, you or a loved one gets cancer, you or someone close to you gets divorced, etc. Overnight, your antennae become super-attuned to this new subject. You notice references to unemployment, pregnancy, cancer, or divorce all over TV, in the movies, in the news, on social media, and in daily conversation. *How did I miss all of this before?* I ask myself. I answer my own question: the subject of MS is no longer hypothetical or abstract; it's intensely personal.

This is where *The West Wing* comes in.

Not too long after I learn I have MS and start taking the wildly expensive medication to treat my disease, I commence streaming the first season of the optimistic political drama on my laptop when I'm doing things like cooking dinner, eating lunch at my desk, or when I simply need a mental distraction. Then I make a realization: *Jed Bartlet, the lead character, has MS too.* Yes, I knew Bartlet had MS when I first watched the show during its initial 1990s-2000s run, but the MS part didn't emotionally register with me. Its mention didn't trigger me. Now, it does. This sudden awareness comes into stark relief when I'm streaming episode twelve and President Bartlet collapses, shattering a Steuben glass water pitcher in the process; he is dizzy and his speech is slurred. Abbey Bartlet's comment, "A fever can be life-threatening," takes on a whole new meaning. This is no longer a fictional story about an erudite New Hampshire governor who becomes president. Although I know I will never be a president, I am now someone with MS.

While I am frantically searching to see if there is a nugget of truth in that fatal fever line, I come across a mention of a *Cleveland Plain Dealer* article quoting the then-president of the National Multiple Sclerosis Society saying that *The West Wing* MS depiction is "a first on network television." It is only after I read the quote, "A fever is no more deadly for people with MS than it is for the general population," that I begin to breathe normally.

Okay, exhale, I think, trying to soothe myself.

But petrifying pop culture MS references seem to crop up regularly.

Several months later, I will see Amy Schumer's *Trainwreck,* a raunchy take-no-prisoners comedy with a big heart. The thing I am not expecting: a storyline about the wheelchair-bound father of Schumer's character, who has been placed in a nursing home alongside residents decades older than him. He needs to be there because his MS symptoms have become so severe that he can no longer live on his own. The cantankerous Mets fan with the foul mouth (**spoiler alert**) hoards his meds and commits suicide. Yeah, that's fun for me, a relatively recently diagnosed MS patient to watch. Intellectually, I understand that everybody's MS evolves differently. There's a range in severity from the kind I have, whose symptoms are not constantly severe (at least for the moment … I'm knocking on wood right now), to the progressive type of MS which worsens unabated. But suicide? After everything I've read about MS *not* being a fatal disease?

Even the darkly provocative Showtime drama of which I become fond in the years following my diagnosis, *The Affair*—a meditation on the impact of an affair on two marriages—has frequent MS references that are likewise gruesome. One of the lead characters, writer-teacher Noah Solloway (Dominic West) reveals to his lover that his teenage years were consumed by taking care of his mother who ... *drumroll please* ... had MS. My mouth falls open after I hear this. This was the last thing I thought I'd be thinking about while watching this program. It was supposed to be a show about how differently everyone sees the world, how the same event can be construed in wildly dissimilar ways by each participant depending on their emotional state, motivation, and point of view. It wasn't supposed to freak me out about MS.

During a subsequent season, Solloway fleshes out the details of his youth spent caring for his mother, telling a therapist: "My sister and I did everything until [my sister] left, so it was just me. Every injection. Every appointment. Giving [her] baths, massaging her legs, changing her diapers." He attributes his mother's early death to MS, saying her life was made too difficult, in the end, by the disease. The character admits he helped her commit suicide.

Again, I consult health websites. As I type "is MS" into the search engine box, Google auto-fills "fatal" for me, as if it is somehow being helpful. In a little over a second, it offers one hundred and ten million results for "is MS fatal." MILLIONS of results. The first one sends readers to the National Multiple Sclerosis Society's frequently asked questions (FAQs). "Is MS fatal?" is the sixth question on the list. The answer is only somewhat satisfying: "Recent research ... indicates that people with MS may live an average of about seven years less than the general population because of disease complications or other medical conditions. ... In some rare instances, there are cases of MS that progress rapidly from disease onset and can be fatal."

This answer leads me to start thinking, *What has happened to the famous people who have had MS? Are there people who have actually died with MS?*

Here's what I find during my research:

I have this vague memory, something about Michelle Obama's father dying in the early 1990s of complications from MS. It's something I kind of remember reading during the 2012 presidential campaign. I locate news stories that confirm my recollection.

Did he die because there were no treatments at that time? I wonder.

This question leads to me figure out that, based on the references in the TV show *The Affair,* the main character's mother would have had MS at around roughly the same time as Michelle Obama's father.

Did people die in the early 1990s because of a lack of available treatments for MS?

Answers don't come easily online. So, I do what I've been trained to do: turn to an expert. Luckily, Dr. Walker allows patients to email him, so I send him some questions and impatiently wait for him to respond. Instead of simply sitting at my laptop refreshing my email account looking for his reply, I want to see what other MS patients have to say.

I buy and devour fellow MS patient Ann Romney's newly released autobiography, *In This Together,* in the hope of learning more about MS. Romney—the wife of the former Massachusetts governor, two-time GOP presidential candidate, and future U.S. senator—detailed her initial 1998 MS diagnosis and her rounds of steroid infusions to combat her symptoms: numbness, muscle spasms, an inability to lift small items, fatigue that flattened her like a panini, and a shakiness on her feet.

"It felt like there was a wildfire raging through me," Romney writes. Following a regimen of steroids and alternative therapies, Romney says she also curtailed her daily schedule to protect her health even as her husband took over the helm of the troubled 2002 Salt Lake City Winter Olympics, when he later became Massachusetts' governor, and then vied for the 2008 Republican presidential nomination.

However, early in the 2012 presidential campaign when Mitt Romney won the Republican nomination, Ann Romney had a severe relapse of MS symptoms, including dizziness, falling, and speech difficulties.

As I am reading Romney's book, news breaks that Jamie-Lynn Sigler—the thirty-four-year-old actress who played Meadow Soprano on HBO's *The Sopranos*—was diagnosed with MS at age twenty and concealed it for years for fear of losing acting roles. In a *People Magazine* interview, she says that now she cannot "walk for a long period of time without resting. I cannot run. ... Stairs? I can do them but they're not the easiest. When I walk, I have to think about every single step, which is annoying and frustrating." Oh, and Sigler is taking the same medication as I am. Romney's book, dovetailed by Sigler's new revelations, offer positive stories demonstrating that you can still live a productive life while under the thumb of an autoimmune disease.

It is around this time when I hear back from my neurologist about my questions involving pop culture depictions of MS treatment, particularly during the early 1990s.

"Treatments first started coming out in the mid-1990s," Dr. Walker, who is the director of an MS center, says in an email. "Patients had to participate in lotteries to get drugs as not enough was available to go around. ... Michelle Obama's father probably did not get care that we are now able to provide for MS patients." Based on his answer, I surmise that the fictional mother on *The Affair* was in a similar situation as Michelle Obama's father. It became really important to me to make a distinction between what happened to them and what was happening to me.

We have disease-modifying medications now. It's not the same, I keep telling myself.

The Romney and Sigler stories indeed provide some solace for me, as does the knowledge that things are different now for MS patients than they were decades ago. Yet Hollywood's depiction of the disease, I am quickly discovering as I revisit *The West Wing* with fresh eyes, consistently leans negative because negative is more dramatic and dramatic equals ratings and ticket sales and clicks.

By the time my streaming of *The West Wing* reaches the sixth season, President Bartlet's MS has become a major plot line once more. During the span of a few days, President Bartlet loses the ability to hold a pen, to walk, to move. He is taken off Air Force One on a stretcher. "Progressive paralysis" the show calls it. He receives infusions (I'm assuming of steroids) during a summit with Chinese leaders. The infusions help President Bartlet regain some mobility during the trip, so much so that he feels strong enough to try to stand on his own in a hotel bathroom, resting his hips on the sink as he brushes his teeth. But he loses his balance, falls forward, twists, and lands on his back on the off-white tile floor, his pants bunched up around his bare ankles. Humiliated. Over the course of a few episodes, President Bartlet transitions from using a wheel-chair, to arm braces, to a cane. At least his mobility issues improve, while his intense fatigue and need for daily naps cause high-level clashes between staffers about when and whether the president should be woken up.

Is it inspiring to imagine that you could still do the job of president while having MS? Absolutely. Right now, I am working hard to push through my own relapsing remitting symptoms while being a writer, an MFA student, and raising three teenagers. But watching the fictional Bartlet struggle, watching him go numb and fall to the floor, hearing his wife say that a fever could kill him ... those scenes cause my imagination to go wild concocting all the possible worst-case scenarios.

Much later, writers for the CBS crime drama *Elementary* will decide to give MS to the girlfriend of a regular character. Soon after she learns she has MS, she breaks up with her police captain beau (Aidan Quinn) because she doesn't want her condition to be a "burden." Confused, the police captain consults a physician friend who, although sympathetic, warns him of only bleak times ahead.

"MS is cruel," says the doctor character, played by Lucy Liu. "The progression is gonna be tough on her, and you. It could take years or months and once the disease relay takes hold, she's gonna need a lot of help."

After the episode ends, the show's official Twitter account sends out this tweet: "What would you do if you were in [the police captain's] shoes?" Translation: Would you dump your girlfriend if she was diagnosed with MS?

I think of my husband, my kids. *Am I going to "get ugly" with MS symptoms? Will I become a burden? Should I give Scott the option of leaving me because the disease could get too hard?*

As my thoughts start to negatively spiral—*This character and this show are contemporary. They're talking about MS patients NOW.*— I take a giant, mental step backward. I must get some perspective.

Am I being too sensitive to this, to what they're saying on a TV show? Am I the only one who feels this way?

Judging by the comments on the National Multiple Sclerosis Society's Facebook page, where the organization posts a video of the MS public service announcement which follows the *Elementary* episode's broadcast, I am not alone in my reaction. Here's a sample of the comments:

"Great to have MS talked about! It would have been better if their description was more accurate! They talked like it was a death sentence. Even went so far as to say there was a timeline for symptoms!"

"I don't watch the show, but I caught the tail end and was shocked and disappointed at how negative the discussion was about MS. They made it sound so fearful."

"I was sad that the discussion on the show was all doom and gloom and how a person with MS would ultimately be debilitated in some form."

During my email correspondence with my neurologist, I ask him about shows and films that depict MS in ways that fail to mention the highly individualized impact of the disease. Dr. Walker writes: "It is really unfortunate that movies and literature utilize these conditions/diagnoses to tell stories. It is a bit like rubbernecking accidents while driving on highways. I bet MS patients have a harder time hearing stories [and watching] movies showing negative MS outcomes since MS patients live with the risk of sudden neurological compromise on essentially a daily basis."

This bugs me for some time, this disease-as-drama proclivity of Hollywood's which affords little to no room for nuance, for authenticity. I speculate on whether cancer patients resent the way cancer is depicted. The way heart attacks and strokes are played out in television shows and films. I can think of dozens of shows and films which cut down characters with cancer or heart ailments. I learn to curtail my over-active imagination and remind myself that these are entertainment.

Entertainment, I tell myself, *just for entertainment. It's not real life.*

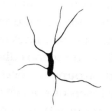

CHAPTER ELEVEN
The New Normal

By November 2014, I have not yet become comfortable with the fact that I'm a grad student. Again. The last time I was a student was the mid-1990s. Bill Clinton was president, grunge was in, I was in my twenties, married, working for a journalism nonprofit, and living in the Washington, D.C. area with Scott and our jumpy cat Plato. Now, I'm in my mid-forties, am still married, have three teenagers, a lazy dog named Max, and am writing from my home office, in my home state, in the greater Boston area. Back in the mid-1990s, Scott and I went to Happy Hours with colleagues (Coronas were super-cheap), regularly visited the national museums (most of which were free, good for twentysomethings on a budget), saw Baltimore Orioles games (my boss would give us tickets), and ate out a lot (lots of barbecue). Nowadays, I find myself mostly at home, writing in my office, and drinking coffee I make with the Keurig. Max sits at my feet. I'm spending my time alternating between voraciously consuming the assigned MFA course readings—the works of Joan Didion, James McBride, Cheryl Strayed, and Susan Orlean—and working on the middle school jazz band book, a process that is going much too sluggishly for my taste. The food we eat is largely made by me (Scott's work schedule has him arriving home by seven or later) and is currently uninspiring. Pizza, subs, or Chinese take-out are thrown in on those nights when I just cannot muster the energy to make dinner.

Pre-MS, I was an impatient multitasker who was up early and got to bed very late and sucked down caffeinated beverages like an addict. I met the deadlines for the variety of places for which I freelanced, tackling pop culture, politics, and parenting. I drove the kids around to soccer, hockey, basketball, and lacrosse, all while teaching college classes.

But in the first few months of my post-MS life, I am growing increasingly frustrated with what seems like the molasses-like speed of everything I do. I am used to having multiple professional irons in the fire. Now, I can only handle a couple, something that will become increasingly more evident when, after I push myself to do too many things for several days without receiving extra hours of rest, I pay the price physically. I become plagued with headaches, find myself too tired to read, and too tired to even watch the news. I require days to recover. This change in my energy level seems as though it has happened overnight, but, perhaps, I just haven't been paying close attention to my waning energy level over the past year, simply attributing it to stress. I think back to the spring when I had a hard time staying awake while helping students edit their newspaper on Thursday evenings even though I was drinking a ton of caffeine. Throw in the fact that I fell asleep during theater performances that were not at all boring, and, the fatigue had simply been increasing over time.

I learn the hard way that my energy reservoir is perpetually in drought conditions and if I don't respect that, I'll have a dangerous deficit.

For example, instead of taking a moderate approach to getting ready to host Thanksgiving 2014, I scour my house in a way that would have made my perfectionist mother proud. I clean the white woodwork throughout the house and remove the fingerprints the boys leave on the door jams when they jump up to strike them with their dirty fingers every time they pass through. I scrub the front of the appliances, the backsplash behind the range-top and become disgusted with how

I've allowed the house to get so dirty. I prepare for overnight guests by cleaning linens and buying some new, soft towels. (The ghost of my mother, who now lives inside my head, is telling me I can't offer rough, old towels to guests.) I shop at multiple specialty grocery stores and wine shops to procure every unique ingredient, wine, and spirit I think we may need, and many we don't. I prepare the side dishes, the desserts, all but the turkey and the stuffing which Scott likes to handle. I create a Thanksgiving playlist and sync up my phone to the wireless speaker. I set up the bar area, arrange the fresh flowers I just bought, lay out the good china, iron the tablecloths and napkins (something I rarely do), then fold those burgundy napkins so they look like flowers blossoming inside the wine glasses, just like Mom used to. In fact, she taught me all of this, how to prepare for a family meal, and how to do it the *right* way. (She was an early fan of all things Martha Stewart and *The Silver Palate Cookbook*.)

For the days following Thanksgiving—an event I cannot enjoy because, by the time the food is on the table, I feel hollowed out from exhaustion—I am in bed. I cannot even work on my grad school assignments or even think about pecking away at another chapter of the book. I lie in bed and argue with myself.

I used to be able to do this stuff, I think. *What the hell?*

As CNN plays on the bedroom TV, it seems too hard to try to even follow what's being said. I begrudgingly realize that things are different now, even though I don't want them to be. It's infuriating. And there's no one who I can hold accountable. No one I can shout at. No one who can do anything to change my current state which does not allow me to act as though I'm fine. Because I am not. I am not fine.

I absolutely do not like this new pace at which I am being forced to live. I do not like that I am taking grad classes on a part-time basis.

identity change!

I should be doing more, my inner, ambitious, pre-MS voice complains.

Dread that I'll eventually suffer from what is described as "cog fog"—a cognitive fog that makes reading, writing, and critical thinking difficult—lingers over me, causing me to question everything I'm trying to do, at least professionally. Worries that fatigue and other symptoms will not allow me to be the kind of mother I want to be to my three kids—two high school sophomores and an eighth grader—are in the forefront of my thoughts. I'm haunted by the high school soccer games I was unable to attend this fall because it was too hot outside and there was no shade in which I could sit. It bothers me that I have already missed several youth hockey games because I was just lying in bed, exhausted. Already, in the past few months I've had to say multiple times, "I can't drive you to your friend's house tonight. I'm sorry. I need to sleep."

I am irate with my own body, for its campaign of self-sabotage, for screwing up my plans, for changing everything, for making me feel as weak and as damaged as my lesion-riddled brain and spinal cord. To the outside world, I am trying to present a face of stoic normalcy. But once I set foot over the threshold of my house, the anger and the frustration return.

This, I realize, *cannot stand.*

I cannot live like this, with all this negativity swirling around inside of me. I cannot just sit around and think about the "what-ifs" of potential, future MS symptoms. Though folks are fond of saying things like, "No one knows the future. Anyone could get hit by a bus tomorrow," for me, the chances of things going south, health-wise, are higher than for the average, previously healthy middle-aged woman.

I decide I need something to inject positivity into my dour attitude. I crave vibrancy, something crackling with life. It isn't that, my personal dramas and demons aside, my household is as placid as still waters. Jonah and Abbey now have their learner's permits. Nothing shakes up a household more than having not one, but *two* teenagers learning how to drive. Jonah's gearing up to travel to Ireland with his high school jazz band over spring vacation in 2015. Casey's busy preparing for his Coming of Age ceremony at our Unitarian Universalist church in April. In the meantime, we're still experiencing "firsts"—first Thanksgiving, first Christmas—without my mother around. Life does not stop nor slow down simply because I have MS or because I am grieving. Life is doggedly indifferent.

While the MFA classes I'm taking spark new creativity and provide an intellectual outlet through which I can dissect what is and has happened to me, I am thirsty for a gleaming distraction from the gloom that adheres to the folds of my brain like barnacles. As impulsively as I did when I enrolled in the MFA program, I seek out a solution in the squirming, yelping form of a puppy. (To my pal Gayle who's chortling at this naiveté: stop laughing.) However, my notion of adopting a physical embodiment of hope and life is not uniformly embraced by the people with whom I live. Scott thinks Max, our five-year-old Havanese-Wheaten terrier mix, is plenty enough canine for us all. Two of the kids think Max will feel slighted and displaced by another dog. Skeptical, I silently wonder if their apprehension is more a reflection of their worries that MS and my writing offer plenty of competition for Mom's limited time and attention. Only one kid agrees that adopting a puppy would allow us to focus on something other than death and illness.

I persist. I press. I lobby. I forward to my family members images of puppies from animal rescue sites that are so sweet your teeth ache just by looking at them. I scan websites in search of a dog, age one or younger, onto whose small shoulders I will place the burden of trying to erase the pall that has become my unwelcome shadow. I become fixated. When I'm not vetting a nightmarish mention of MS from a TV show or movie I just saw, or doing my MFA work, I'm checking the web multiple times a day for available dogs, ready to pounce on a new listing. I eventually win the battle within the household as everyone, reluctantly, consents to moving forward.

I file applications to adopt two different dogs, but not quickly enough. Other dog lovers get their applications in ahead of me. Even in the world of pet adoption I'm moving too slowly. This only prompts me to become more aggressive, to submit applications more quickly. This is what leads to Frasier. Frasier—a slight, bony, brown, tan, black and white two-month-old—is described on the animal shelter site as a mini-Schnauzer mix, *mix* being the key word. The American Kennel Club website tells me that miniature Schnauzers are "friendly, obedient and smart." They're the sixteenth most popular dog breed in the United States, one which has medium energy and a small size. I gaze at the charming photos of mini-Schnauzer puppies, which spark all kinds of gooey maternal feelings. Not a scintilla of negativity can flourish when you're looking at puppies. I envision Frasier curled up alongside Max snoozing in an adorable picture destined to go viral. I see them bounding around our backyard fetching saliva-saturated tennis balls and gnawing on fallen pine tree branches. But that name, Frasier ... it's gotta go.

Already I'm acting possessive, like he's mine, like I have the right to change his name, I think, figuring that's a good sign.

I file the adoption application and then email the listing to Scott. In that order. When I speak with Scott later, I hear the hesitation in his voice. He is so obviously not on board with this, although he is going along with it for my sake, for which I am grateful. I ignore his hesitation. I have my puppy goggles on.

On the last Saturday of January 2015, the whole family, including Max, climbs into the car, drive for a half-hour to shelter in a small Massachusetts town to meet Frasier. He's a floppy-eared little armful with oversized eyes, cow-like pink and tan patches across his soft belly, tender pink paw pads, and a curious jauntiness in his step with lists a bit to the right. Max is unaware that, by virtue of the fact that neither dog is snarling, this little guy is going to come home with us. Without second-guessing, I take Max's neutrality as an endorsement. There is no way we are going home without the tiny furry dude. An hour-plus later, we're in the warmth of our kitchen and Max looks enormous as the newly-renamed Tedy (as in Tedy Bruschi, a former star linebacker for the New England Patriots) cautiously sniffs his new brother's nose, shaggy black and tan ears, his fluffy, feathery tail.

"Te-*dee!*" we coo at him, attempting to orient him to his new name.

It is only after nightfall, which arrives shockingly early in the dead of winter, when I remember with bracing clarity: potty training. I conveniently blotted out of my mind all the work that's required to train a puppy with a teeny bladder to relieve himself outside. I gave no consideration, nada, to sleep or crate training. In my quest to find a puppy heart to heal my own, I blinded myself to reality. It is a shock to my system when Tedy starts whining in his crate, the one into which Scott and I put a cushy dog bed and situated on the floor next to ours. The reality of puppyhood calls with a vengeance at two a.m. when I must carry Tedy outside and over the snow, to which his paws seem rather sensitive. My pajama bottoms untuck themselves from Scott's too-big boots into which I haphazardly shove my feet because they're sitting next to the back door.

Shit! I'm gonna have to do this for weeks.

The cold air bites at my nose and the exposed parts of my neck which is quickly losing its fresh-from-the-blankets warmth. We adopted Max five years ago. In the late summer. We didn't have to do any carrying over snow or bundling him up before taking him outside. As I wait for the petite creature to empty his bladder, I finally grasp what I've done. I'm five years older than when we adopted Max. I now require a lot more sleep and become fatigued much more quickly. Dragging myself out of bed is much harder now than it was then. A few days of getting up in the middle of the night with Tedy is going to render me sleep-deprived, non-functional, and super-cranky. The burden of bringing Tedy outside in the middle of the night will have to fall to Scott. When I put this all together, I finally understand this is one of the reasons he was against this new dog thing in the first place.

⤷

This winter of 2015 is the snowiest New England winter on record. "A six-week-plus snow siege in January-February had parts of New England blowing past all-time records," the Weather Channel says. Over 110 inches of snow are dumped on Boston during the season. In my own backyard, the snow comes up to the hips of my six-foot-tall husband. Icicles form on the roof outside our family room and, in a few weeks, we'll learn they are creating an ice dam which will then start leaking above our brown couch and will collect like a water pouch behind the red paint on the exterior wall. The first full day after we notice the leaking, I will scale the heap of snow on our deck, from which I can reach the roof, and hammer away at the ice dams with so much ferocity that my knuckles start bleeding, leaving pinkish splotches in the snow, something I don't notice until I go inside the house.

Thin little Tedy, who shivers so hard when he's outside that I worry he will detach a retina, is not fond of the snow. Hates it. This makes potty training even more challenging. Lucky for me and for my marriage, Scott never *once* rubs it in my face that I was deluding myself when I said adopting a puppy would bestow cotton candy happiness upon the family. The training process takes longer than it did with Max. It's well into the spring before Tedy gets the hang of it. The kids want no part of the potty training but are more than happy to cuddle with the little beast. I learn I can handle the constant in-and-out of the house business during the daylight hours, when I'm working in my home office, gradually plugging away at *Mr. Clark's Big Band* and my grad work. During the nighttime hours, Scott steps in. I try not to feel guilty about passing the responsibilities off to him so I can sleep. Without that sleep, I'll be useless.

My veterinarian tells me Tedy is most definitely a Jack Russell Terrier (a breed the American Kennel Club describes as "alert, lively, inquisitive" full of "high energy" which is polite code for: a hyperkinetic lunatic). The people at that shelter had no idea what they were talking about when they called him a mini-Schnauzer mix. Maybe he has a bit of Schnauzer, the vet says, but he's mostly Jack Russell. Back when we were looking for Max, Scott researched dog breeds trying to find what he thought was just the "right" one for us. Hyper Jack Russell Terriers were on his "no freakin' way" list. I opt not to tell him right away what the vet says about Tedy's breed, biding my time until the pint-sized fur-ball insinuates himself into my family members' hearts before breaking the news.

Tedy's high-maintenance temperament becomes evident quickly enough when I take him to puppy training classes and the mild-mannered, heavily tattooed and pierced dog trainer is stumped about what I can do to get him to stop with his incessant, ear-piercing barking and his leash yanking. When I attempt to walk Tedy and Max together around the neighborhood, Tedy resists the leash and pulls so far ahead that his collar gags him. He makes a ghastly choking sound that elicits strange looks from passersby, as though I'm abusing my dog, strangling him, or else he has a horrific case of canine TB which I'm now spreading around the neighborhood. He also has a tendency of crossing the sidewalk, zigzagging, back and forth, back and forth. Max the amiable, ambles along, totally low-key, totally "yeah man, whateves," while Tedy is caffeine on legs, attempting to speed-walk while getting his leash tangled up with Max's every two minutes.

The gleaming distraction I was seeking, turns out to be not so much gleaming, but definitely a distraction.

⮑

July 1, 2015.

That's my self-imposed deadline to complete the first full draft of *Mr. Clark's Big Band*. I need something to push me, other than the deadlines for my MFA work. If I want to get this book published before the students, who I shadowed in their middle school music room, graduate from high school in June 2017, I have to get moving.

I tell the band director Jamie that I'll have the first draft done by July 1. I tell a few of my friends about the deadline as well. Once I do that, to me, it's written in stone. I do not want to lose face. I must complete the draft at the same time I work on MFA material and gradually increase my course load.

As spring approaches, I'm feeling emboldened. *I can do this*, I tell myself. *I can finish it.* Suddenly I'm the little blue engine, talking to myself. *A first draft is just that, a first draft. One of many, one that will likely get massively overhauled before the final draft is done. Before I find an agent or a publisher. Before ...* I'm psyching myself out. *Baby steps. I can do this.*

Now that I am focused, I notice that I am writing parts of the book in my head all the time. When I'm showering, I'm coming up with a description. When I'm driving to pick up a kid from the high school, I'm weaving a metaphor and, when I get to stop signs, I scribble them down on scraps of paper. I'm listening to recordings of the middle school jazz band, interspersed with other jazz classics, on repeat to the point where I hear the pieces even when they're not playing. (That's not weird, is it?) When I'm supposed to be sleeping—sleeping is absolutely *vital* to my ability to finish this—my brain (yes, the one with the lesions) won't stop whirring and writing. I am frequently compelled to get up and write things down so, to simplify things, I start to keep a notebook and pen on my nightstand.

I owe the completion of this project not only to the band director, to the Green family whose son Eric's death was the catalyst for this book, to my son Jonah whose rehearsals and grieving I observed first-hand, to the members of the band to whom this year meant so much, but I also owe it to myself. I need to prove to myself that, despite now having MS, I am not beaten.

ᔕ

It's late spring 2015. Tedy is acclimating himself to the house and to his potty training. None of the Tecfidera side effects, the horrifying ones I'd read about, have come to pass. I've adjusted to the medication so well that I no longer have to take the pills with a spoonful of peanut butter to coat and protect my stomach from the pills' contents. My MS symptoms have stabilized. I'm no longer having frequent bouts of light-headedness, nausea, or walk like I recently downed four consecutive shots of tequila. A recent MRI found no new lesions and indicated that none of the existing ones are inflamed. Dr. Walker says this means the Tecfidera is working. Despite the so-called "symptom stability," I continue to experience a sense of numbness on portions of my body which ebb and flow but never completely wane. The zapping sensation up and down my spine when I lower my chin to my chest continues to surprise me every time it occurs. The fatigue comes and goes in its intensity, although I crave my pillow more and more often.

Amid the good news, I feel like I'm waiting for the other shoe to drop. Waiting for the next exacerbation, the next hospitalization. It's just a matter of time, of that I'm sure.

ᔕ

A little more than nine months after being diagnosed, I feel strong enough, confident enough to apply for a teaching job, but only a part-time one, just a tiny advance toward so-called "normalcy," to reclaiming what has been taken from me by illness and circumstance. I find an online listing for a part-time journalism lecturer post at a Boston university to teach students how to interpret the day's news, keeping in mind the context under which the news is gathered. This is perfect as I'm a total news nerd, me with the dead-tree versions of *The New York Times, The Boston Globe* and my local paper, *The MetroWest Daily News* sitting in my driveway every morning. I am a print devotee, love that it leaves inky stains on my fingers, that I can rip an important article out of a page, grab a Sharpie and circle things or write on the paper before leaving it on the kitchen counter for a loved one to read. If I'm feeling play-ful, I make goofy mustaches on photos of people's faces. I'm on Twitter constantly, where I follow many news sites and journalists' accounts. I listen to radio news, read news maga-zines and websites, and have cable news on more frequently than I'd like to admit. I eagerly anticipate political debates the way some folks get excited to watch a big game; I sack out in front of the TV with my laptop and smartphone at the ready. Plus, my student evaluations over my many years of teaching are solid. I'm hoping those help.

Still, I have a nagging sense of insecurity, wondering if this is a massively idiotic thing to do, questioning if I'm ready, if I can handle teaching AND MFA coursework AND finishing the book. These questions, I know, cannot be answered. Dr. Walker cannot tell me if I will get worse and, if I do get worse, when and how. Nobody knows anything. Frustrated by months of having a constrained life, I plunge ahead into the uncer-tainty. What am I waiting for?

During the application process, I am confronted with an online document entitled, "Disability Status: Voluntary Self-Identification of Disability." The university writes, "Because we do business with the government, we must reach out, hire, and provide equal opportunity to qualified people with disabilities. To help us measure how well we are doing, we are asking you to tell us if you have a disability or if you have ever had a disability."

Wait ... what?

"If you already work for us, your answer will not be used against you in any way." However, I didn't already work for the university.

The list of disabilities: blindness, deafness, cancer, diabetes, epilepsy, autism, cerebral palsy, HIV/AIDS, schizophrenia, muscular dystrophy, bipolar disorder, major depression, multiple sclerosis, missing limbs or partially missing limbs, post-traumatic stress disorder, obsessive compulsive disorder, impairments requiring a wheelchair, and intellectual disability. The applicant's choices: check one of the boxes indicating that he or she has or previously had a disability, does not have a disability, or does not wish to answer the question. In order to file a truthful application, I have two options: check "yes" that I have a disability and have them wonder which disability I have, or check "I do not wish to answer" and have them wonder which disability I have. I cannot check "no" because that would be dishonest and morally wrong, however I am not ignorant to the fact that my answer may have an impact on whether I get hired and, because some of these teaching gigs are semester-by-semester, the line that "If you already work with us, your answer will not be used against you in any way" does not seem to apply to me. I have to sign a new contract every semester. I am in a fuzzy gray area here.

The National Multiple Sclerosis Society's website dedicates a lot of verbiage to the employment ramifications of divulging the disease. "The decision to disclose personal medical information in the workplace is a complex one, requiring careful thought and planning," the site says. "Although there may be good reasons to disclose medical information and very specific benefits to doing so, any decision you make today has imme-diate and long-term implications for your employment. It's important to weigh your options carefully before making a decision to disclose—once information is given, it can never be taken back."

What are the dangers of disclosing information you cannot take back? The Society has a page entitled, "Should I Tell?" On one side, the side of disclosing, the Society says:

"Keeping a secret can be stressful and create anxiety.

Once you disclose, you may feel a sense of relief—and find support from people in the workplace.

Disclosing medical information sooner rather than later may provide an opportunity to speak about your MS in a positive light, as opposed to waiting until a problem arises.

It makes it easier to communicate your needs in the event that your condition changes and you need an accommodation."

On the other side of the argument, there are rea-sons the Society suggests considering delaying disclosure:

"Some people have misconceptions about MS and prejudices. Despite your best efforts, they may react negatively toward you, incorrectly viewing you as someone less competent or less able to handle stress.

You could be held back from promotions following disclosure but find it difficult to prove this was due to your MS."

The group's final word on the matter:
"If you are requesting an accommodation or med-ical leave, your employer needs sufficient information about your medical condition or impairment to deter-mine that you have a qualified disability under the

[Americans with Disabilities Act]. This may, in some cases, result in disclosure of your diagnosis.

While it may feel better to disclose information about your medical condition or impairment at this time, it may not be in your best interest in the long run. Special consideration should be paid if you want to take advantage of available legal protections or request an accommodation."

I check "I do not wish to answer," which, in reality, might as well just be a "yes." What kind of people check this box when they *don't* have a disability? People like me, who have or had something but don't want to talk about it outright, are the ones checking this box, the ones whose disabilities aren't openly visible ... as long as I don't have an MS flare-up in front of everybody.

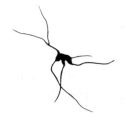

CHAPTER TWELVE
Uhthoff's Phenomenon

I consume lots of coffee to wake me up every morning when all I want to do is sleep. And I get lots of it, sleep. My house isn't as tidy as I'd like it to be. My long, wavy brown hair seems to be permanently bound up in a stretched-out elastic hair-tie atop my head. I've been wearing yoga attire all the time because I can't be bothered to get dressed. We've been eating a lot of take-out, pasta, sandwiches, omelets, and soup, meals that are easy and quick to make. I have been putting my beloved print newspapers straight into the recycling bin because I haven't been able to get to them, despite my best efforts.

But it has been worth it because the first draft of *Mr. Clark's Big Band* ... it is done. Early. I feel like leaping into the air. I want to celebrate. I want to drink champagne and eat decadently. I want to hug everybody. On June 27, 2015—the same day the U.S. Supreme Court rules in favor of gay marriage—I am knocking on Jamie Clark's front door. I have an orange three-ring binder in my arms. It is bursting with the first draft of *Mr. Clark's Big Band*. It's in excess of three hundred-fifty pages. It feels weighty, with expectations, with import.

I hand over the gift of the first draft to Jamie, reminding him that this is simply a draft, to which he says, "Well, yeah. You've written 'draft' all over this!" Which is true. At the top of every page, next to the page number I wrote, "O'Brien – DRAFT." I'm not exactly subtle.

"It's gonna change. A lot," I say, a word of warning lest he get too attached to any particular scene. "I'm going to cut out a lot. I'm going to add some stuff too, but mostly cut. Please tell me if I've got anything wrong in here."

Jamie is giddy. His giddiness is contagious. I can't believe I'm sitting here. On his sofa. With this manuscript. I've finished the first draft. And I have officially been hired to teach journalism at a university in Boston starting in September, at the same time I'll be increasing my MFA course load.

Alongside my optimism, my inner cynic keeps reminding me, *Don't get cocky, kid.*

～

I am enthralled by the painted steps, so clever, so arresting, especially for a book lover like me. The reddish-brown wood on the top of each step is offset by a white painted riser decorated by artsy fonts listing various book categories—home and humor, nautical and nature, teen and middle reader, science fiction and mystery. There are two categories per riser, accompanied by painted images of books. I snap several photos of this staircase, just inside the front door of Edgartown Books on Main Street on Martha's Vineyard.

Bookstores are among my favorite places in the world, along with small movie theaters, brewpubs, local coffee shops, Cape Cod beaches, and Fenway Park. I'm infatuated with the slightly musty, earthy smell of books, by my eagerness to discover the surprises and insights which reside between two covers. The fact that the ink pressed onto the pages of those books may contain thoughts that can change minds, spark new ideas, inspire movements, or elicit visible emotional reactions never fails to fill me with awe. Seeing new writers' books displayed on shelves with signs handwritten by staffers, "Mike recommends this" or "Sheryl recommends this," prompts me to pause and examine the suggested titles.

Edgartown Books is my first stop on my first full day in Martha's Vineyard in July 2015, our family's first vacation since the ill-fated California trip a year ago. The five of us and another family of four, along with their two large golden retrievers Cheyenne and Zoe, are renting a home together in Edgartown for a week. Scott and I are assigned the guest house tucked away in the back of the property, down a little stone path from the "big house," the one in which our pals, Kent and Lise, and our collection of five teenagers will be sleeping. The guest house has recently been renovated and has central air conditioning, something Lise recognizes is important. She knows heat can affect those with MS; her father had MS.

When my family is on board the ferry from Falmouth to Martha's Vineyard, I receive a text from Lise, whose family has already arrived and is settling into the house on High Street. Her text includes a photo of a large, rectangular chalk board on the front of Edgartown Books. "Humorist David Sedaris Aug 1st" a staffer wrote in pink, yellow and purple chalk, with swirls, arrows and flowers floating around the announcement of the appearance of a writer I intensely admire who would be appearing at the Old Whaling Church in Edgartown in a couple of days. "Oh my God!!! I want to go!!!" I text her. "Do you like his stuff? I adore his humor."

"I thought you did," Lise replies.

I never make it to see Sedaris, although I had seen him appear twice at Boston Symphony Hall and nearly pulled stomach muscles because I laughed so hard. A number of things—the weather, heat specifically—conspire against me.

My family arrives at the house after dark. After making sure the kids have something to eat, Scott and I walk six blocks to the restaurant Rockfish to meet Lise and Kent for drinks. There's a light breeze coming off the water, wafting up Main Street. The humidity seems low. I close my eyes and inhale the salty scent of the water. It's the scent of relaxation which I sorely need after the stress of jamming five people's belongings into my battered SUV, of dropping Max and Tedy and all their stuff at a doggie daycare facility, of waiting for the ferry and hoping that during the ride I wouldn't get nauseous. (During the ferry ride, I ply myself with ginger gum and put powder blue motion sickness bands around both my wrists, as I'm apt to get seasick.) Scott and I meet our friends upstairs in the dark wood, mirrored, and windowed bar area. We gather around the right-hand corner of the main bar. The drinks are cold and the laughter feels like a heavy exhale, the kind you make when you have no idea you are holding your breath.

We wake the next day to discover searing sunshine and thick humidity pressing down upon Edgartown. The humidity level is ninety percent. Vacation is ahead of us: Body surfing in the Atlantic, pocketing perfectly shaped scallop shells, eating briny fresh seafood, barreling through an armload of books— read just for entertainment, not work or my MFA classes, and swapping tales and confidences with Kent and Lise under the light of the moon, our wineglasses illuminated by the tiny flames of candles. However, the first thing on my to-do list is to walk the four blocks between our rental house and Edgartown Books. At midday, Scott and I set out for the bookstore. Walking from High Street to South Summer Street, then turning right onto Main Street, we pass large, stately homes, white picket fences, tall hedges, wrought-iron fences painted black. One of those homes is blasting classical music through its open, unscreened windows.

We scale the front stairs to the bookstore, pass beneath the green and white striped awning and enter through the open door. In front of us are those embellished stairs, to the right, the bulk of the bookstore. On the far wall, I see an air conditioning unit. It's working really hard. I feel badly for it, seeing as the heat and humidity pouring through the front door is substantially stronger than the weak Arctic air fighting against it. The air conditioner is losing the fight. Scott and I split up once we enter. I scoop up a Junot Diaz novel, *This is*

How You Lose Her. I pick up Anita Diamant's *The Boston Girl*, a novel by a local author, but put it back down because Lise just bought it the day before and says she'll lend it to me. As I loop around the first floor, I see a large poster promoting an appearance of Ta-Nehisi Coates at the 2015 Martha's Vineyard Book Festival and Author Series on the back wall. Coates had just written *Between the World and Me*, a book that is getting substantial buzz.

I've got to remember to get that, I tell myself.

During this whole time, Scott stands still, in the same location, looking at the same book. He and I have distinctly different ways of shopping. I breeze around haphazardly, a flying insect seemingly without direction, honing in on items of interest, quickly making a decision, then moving on. Scott bores into one item, deeply, which is why it is so maddening for me to try to make any significant purchase with him. He wants to evaluate every option at the cellular level, the polar opposite of my impetuousness. (Prime example: Tedy.) When we were having a sunroom added to our house years ago, he showed me web page after web page of ceiling fans. I gave the thumbs-up to more than six options. On probably the twelfth web page, after we'd already agreed on the style, size, and color of the fan we'd like, he wanted to press on, to exhaust the entirety of our shopping options. Like a sleep-deprived child, I grew irritated, fled the room and told him I trusted his judgment, "Just pick a damned fan. Any fan! I don't care anymore!" On this day in Edgartown Books, I say nothing about his laser-like focus.

"I'm getting this," I say, lifting my Diaz paperback aloft. "You want anything?"

"No," he says, half listening to me.

I pay for my book, but Scott doesn't seem as though he's ready to leave. I mill around, look at some items emblazoned with cover images of famous American book titles when I notice a tingling sensation in my left side, prominently in my left leg and arm. Warmth oozes from my core outward to the surface of my skin as I suddenly feel as though my tank of energy has been aggressively drained.

I need to sit down.

I find a rickety wooden chair not too far from that inefficient air conditioning unit but right in the way of customers who want to walk around the outer edge of the store. I try to make myself smaller, hunch down, push my legs together and my arms inward, worrying that they are judging me, wondering why I'm sitting on my rear end, why I'm so lazy and blocking their way. In all likelihood, no one's judging me. It's probably just me judging myself, annoyed by my need to sit down, by my sudden need to cool off, a need that's escalating exponentially as the seconds pass.

I am silently urging Scott to hurry up, to finish looking at whatever he's looking at, the item he's not planning to buy, when my brain functioning goes haywire. I am starting to feel light-headed, even while I'm sitting here, not exerting myself at all. I'm feeling woozy. All I can think about is cool air, but how many stores in downtown Edgartown have air conditioning? Not many, I'd venture to guess, thinking of the strong Yankee roots of the island.

Aren't New Englanders supposed to be hearty and frugal and into things like sitting in the shade of a tall oak tree to keep cool instead of using air conditioning?

When Scott is finished with his browsing, he finds me. I extend my right arm, a silent plea to help me get to my feet. I hate asking for help, but at this moment I need it. My limbs aren't moving like they should. I see stars across my field of vision when I, with tremendous difficulty, get to my feet. Moments after we emerge from the bookstore, into the moisture-rich air, things quickly worsen. I am not at all well. I have the look of a person who has over-imbibed as dizziness and instability overcome me. My vision blurs, my stomach lurches. I think I'm going to vomit. I need to get out of this heat and humidity but don't want my MS to make Scott prematurely go back to the house. I see a clothing store not too far away on the corner with its doors closed.

It must have air conditioning, I think. "Let's go there," I say, trying not to let on how badly I feel, although I am leaning on him pretty hard.

Once inside the store, I realize this is fruitless. There are no chairs onto which I can collapse. The shelving units don't look like they can hold me up. I need to lie down. I worry I'll faint onto the sidewalk and cause another scene like that one in Santa Monica where I looked like I had passed out on the grass. Or perhaps I'll start getting sick to my stomach like I did at the Hollywood Bowl. How I look to others worries me. I worry they'll think I'm drunk or lazy or incompetent or overly sensitive as they see me wilting in the heat and humidity. I worry about inconveniencing those around me, ruining their evenings, their vacations, their dinners, their birthday celebrations, their lives with all these MS-related needs. I worry about being this burden, this burden on the sidewalk.

I thought I was getting better, that I was stable, I think, not immediately factoring in how sensitive to the heat my multiple sclerosis has made me, despite the reading I have done on the subject.

After the debacle on Main Street, I am under a house arrest of sorts, holed up in the air-conditioned guest house, to cool off, rest, and regain my equilibrium. While I'm lying on the bed in the middle of the day feeling irritated and lonely, I research heat sensitivity on my smartphone and everybody else is enjoying the beach. I read up on Uhthoff's Phenomenon, which is not really a phenomenon so much as a life obstacle. I learn that this nineteenth century German doctor, Wilhelm Uhthoff, discovered that patients with multiple sclerosis experience a temporary flare-up of symptoms of their disease when they are overheated. When an MS patient is too hot and her symptoms resurface—like blurry vision, mobility, nausea, and balance issues—it's called Uhthoff's Syndrome (or Uhthoff's Phenomenon or, occasionally, Uhthoff's Sign).

Long before the advent of MRIs, which allow neurologists to spot the lesions left behind by multiple sclerosis' assaults on brain and spinal nerves, doctors, inspired by Dr. Uhthoff, utilized what they called the "hot bath test" as a diagnostic tool. "A person suspected of having MS was immersed in a hot tub of water," the National Multiple Sclerosis Society's website says. "The appearance of neurological symptoms or their worsening was taken as evidence the person has MS." (When I discuss this old diagnostic approach with Dr. Walker, he calls it "horrendous.") Walking around in heat and humidity, spending time in an overheated room, and just getting too hot can result in the appearance of temporary symptoms that mimic an MS attack. This is what happened to me at the bookstore. Even "a very slight elevation in core body temperature" can "impair the ability of a demyelinated nerve to conduct electrical impulses," the Multiple Sclerosis Society says.

Not all MS patients experience heat sensitivity, Dr. Walker tells me later. "What it represents is that you have the axons, the neurons ... the machinery, the electrical parts, but you don't have the myelin in that one area and it shorts out when you're overheated or stressed."

No one has figured out how to combat this. Avoiding the heat and humidity is the only guidance MS patients with heat sensitivity are given, that and wearing hideous "cooling" clothing items. Before leaving for Martha's Vineyard, I had asked Dr. Walker for his advice about what I should do if I get too hot while sitting on the beach. He scrunched his face and looked at me strangely. "You just jump in the water!" he said, as if I am going to spend an entire day sitting in the water like a saturated sponge. It was not a helpful piece of advice.

After several hours inside the vacation rental's guest house, Scott and I—communicating via text—eventually figure out how to navigate this heat sensitivity, at least for the week we're in Martha's Vineyard. I will avoid going to hot and humid places during the day, avoid locales where there is no air conditioning into which I can seek relief. I will only join the rest of my family and friends at the beach after five p.m., when the sun isn't strong and after the heat has (hopefully) diminished. On the days when it remains hot after five, I will have to repeatedly take dips in the water and avidly stay out of the sun. Worst case: I'll have someone drive me back to the house if I become sick. It doesn't please me, this notion that, for the rest of my life, I won't be able to sit on the beach with everyone else until early evening, like I'm permanently grounded, but I really have no other option.

The incident at the bookstore teaches me that heat is my Kryptonite. It goes beyond skipping a day at the beach so I don't become a literal hot mess. I realize that this heat sensitivity affects many aspects of my life. Weeks after the Martha's Vineyard trip, I have to pass up attending several Red Sox games—tickets for games I purchased and gave to Scott as Christmas gifts with the hope he'd ask me to accompany him— when it is predicted to be steamy late into the night. I cannot attend outdoor concerts or festivals or summer barbecues if it's going to be hot or humid outside and there's no refuge.

When we get home from vacation, I turn the house into a refrigerator for the rest of the summer to avoid triggering MS symptoms. To keep me lucid, upright, and not nauseous, the temperature is set for the maximum of seventy-three degrees, although seventy is better. To the rest of the family, this is freezing, especially in the month of August. And they're starting to gripe about it.

On a humid, late August morning in 2015, Jonah—an every-rib-poking-through-the-skin kind of skinny—stomps out of his bedroom wearing two long-sleeved T-shirts and fuzzy pajama bottoms. His room, he declares, is "like a freezer."

Sitting at the kitchen table, sipping my iced coffee while wearing shorts and a short-sleeved T-shirt, I shrug.

Of course he's cold. He's got no body fat, I think but don't say out loud.

But his complaints about being freezing, about having to layer on a comforter and an extra blanket when he sleeps, are quickly echoed by Abbey and Casey, both of whom dress for a winter night's slumber in August. The coolness of the over-worked air conditioner doesn't chill me as it does them. Without mentioning the perimenopausal hot flashes I've recently begun to experience, I explain to them that the cold keeps my head clear (something with which I'm guessing they'd quibble), prevents me from getting dizzy, from seeing spots, from crippling nausea, from my knees buckling. But, a year after my MS diagnosis, I look at my heavily layered teens and admit that this highly air-conditioned life is starting to become a problem, albeit a problem with no real alternative. If I don't jack up the AC, I will be a listless puddle. They're just going to have to get bigger blankets.

Being at home, where I control the temperature is one thing. Being out of the house in situations where I have no control over the temperature is another. I am now developing a fear of being trapped in an overheated situation that could melt me like a Popsicle. Meteorologists are becoming my soothsayers as their weather forecasts tell me if I need to tuck an ice pack, or several, into an insulated bag tucked into my purse so I can watch my elder son perform during Pops Night in the stuffy high school. They tell me how to prepare for an end-of-the-season banquet for the high school track team inside that same gymnasium when I apply a series of icy cans of soda to my neck and face as my husband and friends con-tinuously replenish my supply of chilled cans so I don't have to leave the banquet because I'm succumbing to the heat.

⌒

Eighteen months ago, I considered my freshly retired

father a gourmet chef whose food I had enjoyed for many years. In the mid-1980s, when Mom started coming home late from work managing two wine and liquor shops, Dad, a liquor salesman with a more flexible schedule, took it upon himself to establish his culinary chops by taking the voluminous gastronomic knowledge my mother gave him and expanding upon it. As his talent and enthusiasm for cooking grew, people would lavish his dishes with praise. (If Mom was around to hear the compliment, she was quick to chime in with an, "*I* taught him that.")

Dad's approach to cooking was way different than Mom's. For him, it was all about vast quantities of food eaten with gusto. If you invited him to a college tailgate party, to a family barbecue, to a backyard birthday party, or to an Easter brunch at your house, he loved nothing more than to contribute by bringing a portable feast along with him, regardless of what the hosts had prepared. He was apt to haul the thick metal pot my mother got from her mother—who got it from her mother who got it in her hometown in Spain—and fill it with chili, thick with hunks of sirloin, sautéed onions and peppers, and spicy Italian sausage. He'd also have a Crock Pot of homemade baked beans. Oftentimes, he'd offer to roast a turkey breast to go "on the side" of whatever main course we were serving at an event. "Just in case people feel like having turkey," he'd say, as if it was somehow commonplace to bring a roasted turkey breast, chili, and gallons of baked beans to a children's hamburgers-and-hot dogs birthday party. Or perhaps, he'd suggest, we'd be interested in a Bolognese dish in a forty-eight-quart bowl? Or a heaping platter of homemade Buffalo wings, extra hot (because if you don't sweat when you eat them, you're doing it wrong)?

The food my father brought to gatherings was not at all like the delicate, camera-ready dishes favored by Mom, except maybe for the lobster bisque he loved to make, with a touch of cognac. Mom saw cooking less as a source of joy than as an art form, both the food and its presentation. Her best-of-the-best meals looked as though they sprung to life from the glossy pages of a food magazine, laid out on festively dressed tables, accompanied by tasteful seasonable decorations and place cards. Dad's cooking—which began with lowly boiled hot dogs cushioned in soft J.J. Nissen rolls, B&M baked beans from a can, with a side of greasy State Line Potato Chips piled onto a paper plate and consumed in front of a M*A*S*H repeat, as long as Sean and I didn't tell Mom we'd eaten in front of the TV—was all about volume and comfort; bring on the paper plates and napkins, no need to stand on ceremony.

After Sean and I moved out of the family home and into apartments of our own, Dad continued to spend his free time preparing elaborate meals and dishes. Filet mignon that he picked out at the Ye Olde Butcher Shoppe on North Boulevard after consulting with the butcher, because the guy knows his cuts of meat. Hearty beef stews with an infusion of Burgundy and large chunks of Yukon Gold potatoes. Chorizo-filled Portuguese soup, made in accordance with the recipe from The Moors in Provincetown, the inn/restaurant where my parents stayed on their honeymoon in 1968. He'd bring these heaping helpings of his latest endeavors to my house and to my brother's house, love in a battered metal pot.

Dad frequently reminisced about the days when Scott, I, and several of our college friends, would have a quick dinner at his house before leaving to attend college basketball games during winter breaks. It gave Dad so much satisfaction to watch us all scarf down the food. "Who wants more?" Dad would ask, his ladle poised above a pot of chili as we inhaled the food. "Come on! Come on! Come on! You guys can eat more than *that*!" He'd say this even after several of us had additional helpings. Mom would be noticeably irritated about our dining-and-dashing in order to make the tip-off, as we left crumbs, dirty dishes, and hasty "goodbyes" in our wake, but it didn't bother Dad a bit, as his pleasure came from watching us gorge ourselves on his creations.

That seems like a very long time ago.

A mere eighteen months ago, Dad's focus narrowed from bringing tons of food to my house or Sean's house, from creating meals his grandkids would adore, to filling one belly: my mother's. All of the labor, the flourish, the abundance he whipped up in the kitchen, it was for her. He was trying to stuff her with nourishment when she didn't want to eat, when she couldn't eat because the chemo and the growing tumor in her abdomen had obliterated her appetite. Dad would frequently call me from someplace in the house where it sounded echoey, like he was crouching behind something. He would hoarsely whisper into the phone: "She won't eat *anything*. I made her steak tonight and she didn't eat any of it. Didn't even taste it. Said her stomach was bothering her." His voice was a mixture of disappointment with the strong tang of fear. "So I made her chicken soup, but she wouldn't eat that either. Just wanted tea."

When Dad wasn't around, Mom would make her own clandestine calls. "Your father keeps making these big meals for me and I'm just not hungry," she would say. "I pretend to take a bite, but he keeps saying his feelings are hurt."

Nowadays though, he doesn't cook at all. Even when we beg him to do so.

"Hey Dad, can you make something to bring to Christmas?" I asked him before our first Christmas since Mom died. He agreed and showed up with a bag of frozen shrimp and a raw roast from the grocery store.

In July 2015, he shocks us by renting a house on Lake Winnipesaukee in Meredith, New Hampshire. It's a place where his parents used to take him and his brother when they were young, a place where nostalgia is like a rip current. While Scott, the kids and I join him for a weekend, Abbey decides to try to resuscitate his dormant culinary skills, to breathe new life into them. She asks him to show her cooking techniques, the way Grandma taught him. Before we arrive, Abbey asks me if I think getting him to cook with her will make him happy.

"I don't know sweetie," I say, keeping my doubts to myself.

They decide to make lasagna together, one of Dad's exceptional dishes. Abbey asks him to accompany her to the market to buy the ingredients. Once the duo returns to the lake-side house, she plays upbeat music on her phone and chatters away to fill the silences. Her aching desperation to get the Grandpa she once knew back is palpable. He participates somewhat half-heartedly in the cooking process, often sits on a stool and watches her work, occasionally chiming in, but mostly saying very little. The result of their efforts: a densely layered lasagna that is too large for its own pan. It is willingly gobbled up by my three teens, but the enthusiasm Dad once held for watching people eating what he has made just isn't there anymore. He barely eats any of his slice.

In this moment, I realize I'm not the only one who's numb.

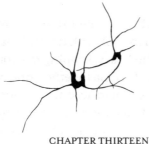

CHAPTER THIRTEEN
Coatless in Quincy Market

It is almost two inches long and half as wide. It's as black as a dog's nose. It's shiny and smooth, although pocked with tiny holes that can't be immediately felt by my fingertips. I have no idea what kind of stone it is, but I do know where it came from: Katama Beach on Martha's Vineyard, where my family spent time a few weeks ago, me only visiting after five o'clock to avoid any dramatic, heat-related pseudo-flares.

I find the stone resting atop a slightly crinkled piece of canary yellow lined paper on my desk: *Here is a worry stone that you can take to school with you. Every time you look at it you can think of how much I love and support you. Love, Abbey.*

It is hours before I would be heading into the unknown after a summer of I'd-rather-forgets. Teaching is certainly not new to me as I've only been away from a university classroom for a year. What *is* new is stepping in front of students as someone who has multiple sclerosis. Every experience in a new arena in my post-diagnosis life now seems potentially precarious, seeing that I cannot predict the conditions in which I'll be working, therefore cannot envision how my body will react. Starting a new job in an unfamiliar place, coupled with having an unpredictable disease, stokes the embers of my always-burning anxiety. And that anxiety must have been evident to everybody in the house, thus the gift of the worry stone.

My chief concern: will the classroom be too hot for me and provoke a physical reaction, the kind I just experienced on vacation? If I tell my new employers that I have MS, will that jeopardize my future there? I'd really like my teaching abilities to speak for themselves and for MS to be a non-issue. That's what I'd really like. I don't know if I'll get my wish.

The worry stone from my seventeen-year-old daughter, left next to my first-day-of-class lesson plan, becomes my talisman, one that gives me courage because I know she has faith (even if I don't) that things will work out. I clutch it tightly during the commute into Boston. I blast the air conditioning in my car—attempting to pre-freeze myself on this sticky September afternoon—and try not to dwell on worst-case scenarios. The stone, growing hot in my sweaty palm, starts to smell of lavender as the French hand cream I used earlier—picked specifically because the scent is supposed to soothe—is absorbed into its surface.

My thumb presses into its unforgiving hardness. I caress it methodically with the pad of my thumb.

Back and forth.

Back and forth.

A solitary prayer bead.

No matter how hard I press into it, it will not give. It will remain solid. No matter what happens.

⌐

I step into a veritable sauna of a university classroom on the first day of the semester. There are no windows here as we're in the basement which should, in theory, be cool. It's not. There is no way to control the temperature.

This is going to be interesting.

I take this like the challenge it is. Luckily, I wore a sleeveless summer dress and piled my long, thick brown hair atop my head. Getting ready for class becomes a strategic venture as I don light clothing and bring ice packs—to clandestinely press into my hands and against my neck—into insulated lunch bags.

I bring an icy drink with me to sip and to chill my hands. It will be rare for me, throughout the semester, to let my heavy hair rest on my neck.

As fall becomes winter, the situation inside this overheated room gets worse after the heating system kicks on in earnest. I am fearful, at every single class meeting of the semester, about the impact of the heat, concerned I'll be felled, mid-sentence during a discussion about cable news coverage of a 2015 presidential primary debate, that one of the many symptoms which now manifest themselves when I'm overheated will overtake me. I continue to wear thin layers even after the first frost. I replenish my stock of all things sleeveless—at least summer dresses are now on sale—and wear them, regardless of the outside temperature. I continue buying ice coffee to hold against my face when I turn away from the class if I'm getting too warm. In what seems like a minor miracle, I'm able to get through the semester without incident.

What I cannot plan for, what the meteorologists cannot help with, are unpredictable circumstances involving heat inside of buildings during the winter. On a December 2015 evening, my family visits the Quincy Market food court in Boston. You'd think that Boston, in the winter, would be no big deal for someone with heat sensitivity. You'd think that wouldn't you. Except for one factor I haven't considered: overzealous furnaces. Entering that bustling marketplace, where the heat is cranked and the customers' heavy coats emit steaminess into the stuffy air, my knees weaken, I see spots in my vision, and curl over with nausea. I tell Scott and the kids I will wait for them outside, where I stand between white pillars on the concrete steps, in just a thin shirt and jeans in thirty-degree weather—my coat, scarf, hat, gloves, and sweater in a heap on the sidewalk. Because of the heat, Scott and the kids agree to eat our dinner outside by my side, on the steps of Quincy Market. Our breath makes little clouds in front of our faces.

After I created a July 1, 2015 deadline for me to complete the first draft of *Mr. Clark's Big Band*, I realize I need to give myself another one. By January 1, 2016, I want to have the manuscript in good enough shape to start shopping it around to publishers and/or literary agents. If I want the students who were middle school jazz musicians when I observed them in 2012-2013 to see this book published before they graduate from high school, I need to create some parameters. My mother's illness and death, my father's hospitalization, my own illness, all of these things threw my original plans for this book out of whack. As I now look at the calendar and work backward to see when I need to get someone to agree to publish this so the kids about whom I wrote have this book in their hands before graduation, I start to get panicky.

My top priority is getting this manuscript in publishable shape. The part that comes after that, the getting it published part, is beyond my control. I will be at the whim of the marketplace, whatever's hot, whoever happens to be moved by my pitch letter, and how fast they respond. But to make a June 2017 publishing deadline—when Eric Green's classmates, including my twins, Jonah and Abbey, graduate from high school—I need to step it up. I just hope my body—my damaged brain and spinal cord—will not betray me.

Between now and then, I need to ruthlessly edit this thing, to pare it down to the essence of what's important. In the first draft, I wrote about nearly everything I witnessed that had any literary value. Unfortunately, upon reading it through, I realize a significant portion of the scenes do not really advance the story; they weigh it down. Several friends who read the first draft and give me their input, tell me the first part of the book is a bit drawn out. In response, I stiffen my spine, pull out the editing knife, and start cutting. Although this is a painful process—because I struggled to craft the right phrases, locate the precisely-correct words for every scene in the first draft—I must do what's best for the project. Additionally, I'm workshopping sections of the manuscript in my MFA classes— have been since I entered the program—and am benefitting from their advice as well.

January 1, 2016 seems doable, right? I ask myself.

In December 2015, after I complete the first semester of post-MS diagnosis teaching—correct all the final papers, compute and submit the final grades for forty-nine students, *after* I submit my own MFA projects for the three courses I'm now taking as a full-time student, *after* I buy Christmas presents for my two high school juniors and one high school fresh- man—I spend an entire weekend purging my manuscript of everything that slows it down.

Right about now, I could really use a peaceful yoga class, but in September I had to give up yoga after I realized I simply cannot be a full-time student, edit the book, teach part-time, AND make a regular yoga practice. I am greedily seizing every moment of sleep I can. I'm not going out at night or on the weekends. I am going to sleep early and stay in bed as long as possible in an effort to keep me going. Sleep is my fuel. The yoga, regardless of how great everyone (including Dr. Walker) says it is for MS patients, will have to wait. In December, Scott is pushing hard for me to return to yoga, as are the kids who think I'm nicer and more patient when I'm exercising. (They're right.) I know they mean well, but I just cannot do it. I cannot fit anything else into my world. Yes, I know that yoga helps manage stress, but there are only so many hours in the day.

What do these people want from me?

꡷

Shortly after I got my diagnosis, I started following Twitter accounts written by MS advocacy groups, MS support groups, and MS patients. Amid the news updates, the witty quips about

Game of Thrones developments, the lamentations of Red Sox fans when the team fares poorly, I am reminded of my multiple sclerosis whenever I check Twitter. The takeaway I derive from reading these social media feeds: *You could become very sick, become disabled ... any day now.* I know I have been lucky thus far in my MS experience. Things could be much worse, and yet ...

One day I click on a tweet from an MS support group which leads me to a first-person essay about a woman who has multiple sclerosis. She writes: "I am not new to MS but am new to being officially 'disabled.' After more than a decade without symptoms following initial diagnosis ... my MS worsened and I could no longer perform my stressful job." She continues saying she feels adrift without her work identity and asks for advice. I read her essay. Then re-read it.

This leads me down the kind of internet rabbit hole into which people sometimes find themselves, clicking on one article, only to have another on the same topic suggested for your reading pleasure. I stumble upon another essay, written by a woman named Linda Chavers in an online magazine called *Dame.* The title: "34 Things I Wish Multiple Sclerosis Hadn't Shown Me." Chavers is turning thirty-three and is reflecting on the nine years she has spent dealing with this incurable autoimmune disease. "This is not an essay about being single in your thirties," she writes. "This is an essay about the ugliness of sick. About the discoveries it forces upon you."

I freeze for a few seconds and ponder whether I should proceed any further, whether reading this will terrify me. I can't help myself. I keep reading. Her voice is compelling. Bit by bit, Chavers describes losing parts of herself, her ability to wear heels, her ability to partake in group exercise classes which take place in studios that are too warm. Four years post-diagnosis, she starts limping on her left side which consequently weakens. At seven years, "I cannot walk more than half a mile before collapsing. I can no longer run, period."

The part that hits me hardest is number twenty-eight on her list: "There's a particular sense of urgency to my writing. Cognitive dysfunction and decline are signatures of MS and I don't know if or when these will start, if they haven't already. Writing is a way I tell the world I was here, I mattered."

I am now petrified.

⟅⟆

While having a chronic and unpredictable disease is hard for the patient, it's unbelievably frustrating for that patient's family. In my case, as we slide into 2016, I start to take stock of how MS has changed life for my family, for Scott, Abbey, Jonah, and Casey. It has not changed for the better, at least from my perspective. I am not the wife and mother I wish I could be, the one I used to be.

Although I look perfectly healthy to the outside world, these four people know the truth. They see me when I hit the wall, fatigue-wise, when my face goes several shades paler than it normally is and I retreat to my bed at six p.m., unable to move, but insistent that I can still teach, edit the manuscript, and finish my MFA all simultaneously. They are on the unfortunate receiving end of my venting over minute, daily life irritants, like when I have to wash mountains of dishes because the pile explodes out of the sink and snakes its way along the counters. They watch as I push everything else to the side—including, on occasion, dinners, and attending extra-curricular kids' activities—in order to whip the manuscript *Mr. Clark's Big Band* into shape and send it out to agents and publishers, which I've just started doing in the beginning of 2016, just like they see the aftermath of such efforts, the lethargy the fatigue forces upon me.

When I become overwhelmed with that fatigue when I'm outside of the house, I become convinced that, to passersby, I seem like a temperamental, spoiled brat, vacillating between snarling at my loved ones and collapsing upon a chair with a huff. Occasionally, I press my weary body into a doorjamb to keep me from literally sliding to the floor. It's not a good look. I am not in a particularly good place right now.

I am teaching another journalism class in the spring semester at the university, after having received excellent teaching reviews from the fall. I have a slate of nearly fifty students again. The world outside of the classroom is exceedingly generous in providing us ample material to analyze, what with the 2016 presidential primary campaign in full gear. Every day, sometimes multiple times a day, something new and unprecedented happens at the intersection of news and politics that it's becoming difficult to keep up with it all. But keep up I must in order to fulfill my charge of guiding my students in the educated interpretations of the daily news. This means keeping current, constantly. I am falling asleep at night with CNN on the TV in my bedroom, waking up in the morning and turning it on again while I lie in bed and scroll through Twitter before getting up to go read the newspapers that Scott has brought in from the driveway and placed on the kitchen counter for me.

To try to get a handle on my life, the one, several months ago, about which I was complaining because it was moving too slowly for my pre-MS mind to accept. I start assigning my tasks specific days of the week so I can tackle my fast-flowing spigot of to-do items. On Mondays, I do class prep and grade papers. On Tuesdays, I work on MFA assignments in the morning and teach class in the afternoon. On Wednesdays, I work on *Mr. Clark's Big Band*. On Thursdays, I do class prep and more MFA work. On Friday afternoons, I teach. On the weekends, I crumple into a ball on a sofa, marshaling only the energy to read the newspapers, especially the Sunday editions, because I MUST keep current.

What was I thinking? This pace is unsustainable, I tell myself, surveying, with great dissatisfaction, how stressed out I am, how I keep missing things in my personal life, how I feel as though I'm constantly running behind. It's feast or famine. Although, intellectually, I realize this pace is not working for me, emotionally, I am frustrated that it feels so difficult. I pray I have not set myself up for a massive failure.

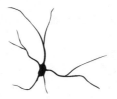

CHAPTER FOURTEEN
Meltdown in the London Rain

Scott wants to plan a family get-away for the summer of 2016. To someplace we've never been. Someplace where it won't be too hot or humid in early-June. Someplace that will mentally take me out of the whole book business, out of my MFA coursework. He envisions an odyssey that will be festive, not just for him and for me, but for our three kids.

England.

London, to be specific. London in the late spring, before it gets too hot for me.

Neither Scott nor I have been overseas, other than a trip to Aruba for our honeymoon in 1992, and a family road trip to Montreal and Quebec in 2010. Jonah went to Ireland last year with his high school jazz ensemble. Abbey is slated to spend her 2016 spring vacation in France as part of the high school's student exchange program, (We hosted a French student, Marianne, at our house for two weeks in the fall of 2015.)

As Scott did with our California trip two years ago, he starts researching and planning what he's billing as our "last big family vacation" before Abbey and Jonah go to college. I can offer him no assistance as I can focus on nothing other than my own stack of tasks. This is going to be our resident fixer's show and we're going to be following his directions, hit all our marks.

We take off from Boston's Logan Airport in June 2016 with Scott's plans in hand, with the spring 2016 semester of my journalism class and my MFA classes over, with the kids' classes done for the summer, and with no publisher or agent for *Mr. Clark's Big Band*.

⤐

A few days into our trip, the fatigue strikes. We have been touring hot spots in London for days without incident. Tower of London. Parliament. Westminster Abbey. The British Museum. Trafalgar Square. Buckingham Palace. But by late lunchtime, one day midway through the English odyssey, lethargy overcomes me, as if I've been unplugged. I cannot articulate what is happening to me as it's happening, I only know that I need food and rest. Immediately. My level of patience is rapidly reduced to that of a toddler's as I feel as though my circuiting is misfiring.

If this was a movie, this is what the script would look like when we enter a very fancy restaurant for high tea after having toured the Churchill World War II bunker all morning:

SCOTT
(*Looking at a menu on a stand inside the swanky, upscale restaurant, where it doesn't look as though are many food options the kids will like.*)
So, what do you think? Want to eat here?
Have you looked at the menu?

Meredith gives a cursory glance in the direction of the menu.

MEREDITH
No. ... I don't know. ... Whatever. (*Refuses to explain*)

SCOTT
(*A questioning look on his face*)
Um, why? Do you see anything you could eat?

Meredith glances at the menu again, not really reading it.

MEREDITH
The kids won't eat this.
(Pauses a beat. Frowns, wrinkles brow. Knows it's not about what the kids will eat. Or what she, the dairy-allergy sufferer, can eat.)
I need to sit down. You guys decide. I don't care.

ABBEY
(Playing peacemaker)
Mom, there are things here we'll eat, some things you can eat too.
(Referring to her mom's dairy allergy)

Meredith blankly stares, shrugs shoulders while her eyes seek out a place to sit. There is no place to sit. She fights the urge to lie down on the floor where she's standing.

CASEY
(Normally the always-hungry picky eater, also playing the role of peacemaker)
Well ... maybe we could have this.
(Points to an item on the menu)

SCOTT
(In fix-it mode)
Want me to ask if they have dairy-free options?

Not hearing a response, Scott flags down a restaurant employee to ask menu questions, while Meredith retreats to a doorway and awkwardly leans against it, facing away from Scott.

ABBEY
(Rubs her mother's back and talks to her softly, as one would do with a child)

UNCOMFORTABLY NUMB
177

You okay Mom? Dad's trying to find out what you can eat.

Meredith does not respond. She can't seem to access the language necessary to explain, doesn't even understand the ferocious microburst change in mood and energy that has overwhelmed her. Scott, walking with a sense of urgency, approaches Meredith and Abbey.
The two boys trail along in his wake.

SCOTT
There are things you can eat. I asked. The kids said there are things they're willing to have. Do you want to eat here, or do you want to go someplace else?

MEREDITH
(*Angry, more with herself, with her lack of explanation, comprehension*)
I just want to go back to the hotel!

Scott looks outside. It's now absolutely pouring.
Sheets of liquid. No cabs in sight.

SCOTT
Well why don't we wait here? We could ...

MEREDITH
... I want to go back to the hotel!

Tears start to stream down her face. She darts outside to the steps, then, upon feeling the deluge of rain on her face, backtracks to stand beneath the tiny awning. Meredith starts sobbing. She feels trapped and idiotic. Scott, who followed her outside then stood on the threshold, is, understandably, annoyed. The kids, unsure about what's really happening, look back and forth from mother to father.

It's an understatement to say I do not cover myself in glory on this afternoon. I am tangled up inside myself, in a web of self-loathing for feeling immobilized by inertia that strikes with the suddenness of lightning. My voice is choked off, strangled by my emotional paralysis. Had I been able to think rationally, I would have realized that a) I am hungry b) I am pushing myself to do too much while getting insufficient rest but am too stubborn to admit this because I don't want to be a stick-in-the-mud and prevent my family from enjoying this adventure and c) if I get some rest, I will feel better.

Scott is always trying to read me, to figure out what is going on, and act based on his independent assessment. He is my self-appointed caretaker and is trying to make everyone happy, but I am a source of frustration at which he cannot lash out. Jonah, Casey, and Abbey, meanwhile, just want peace. As well as something to eat. Scott—who continues to feel guilty about how we handled my MS exacerbation during the LA trip, and about the fact that I spent the bulk of last summer on Martha's Vineyard holed up inside an air-conditioned guest house while everyone else was at the beach—wants to care for me, to care for all of us. He has prearranged every aspect of our jaunt very carefully, around my MS, trying to get us all to head back to the hotel early, and not stuffing too many events into a single day. He is really trying, and for that, I am also angry. I don't want him to have to take care of me. I feel like I'm back to square one, fighting against my disease again, rebuffing the necessity of special treatment.

Ultimately, I calm down and the afternoon markedly improves when we find a cab and grab a bite to eat at a casual restaurant a block away from the hotel at which we've already eaten so we know everyone would find an acceptable food choice. (Scott's bloody brilliant suggestion.) After everyone's hunger is satiated, we go back to the hotel and I get some rest. Reflecting on my meltdown in the London rain, I acknowledge to myself that I could have avoided all this drama had I not been slowly stewing in resentment about having to take breaks, about me having to avoid scaling stairs (which meant not being able to enjoy several historic landmarks accessible only by stairs, like the inside of a tower at the Tower of London or later, buildings at Oxford University), and having to go to bed early like a retiree. Scott and the kids have been absolutely accepting of the adjustments made to the trip to accommodate me, at least they said they were. I am the problem. As far as I've come in trying to accept changes to my life because of this disease, acceptance does not proceed in a straight line.

⌐

Once we get home from England, I receive good news. An independent publisher is willing to publish *Mr. Clark's Big Band* in May 2017.

My book will be published! I shout inside my head when I receive the publishing agreement via email. I am on a high, having finally, after six months of "no's" and finally getting a "yes." But the high wanes once I begin to think about all the work ahead of me including last-minute editing, public relations, and all the behind-the-scenes work that goes into publishing.

Am I going to hit an MS wall? I ask myself again, the same question that continues to pop up, repeatedly, whenever I step into another adventure as an MS patient. Pre-MS this would be stressful but totally doable, given the right amount of caffeine. But things have changed.

Will I also be able to finish my MFA and write a thesis, now that I'm getting Mr. Clark's Big Band *published?* Since entering grad school, I have changed my mind about my thesis. Instead of submitting *Mr. Clark's Big Band*, I decided to create a new thesis, one that would have to be written and submitted in less than a year. Why? Because I'm an idiot. The publication date for *Mr. Clark's* is weeks before I am to finish my MFA program and a month before Abbey and Jonah graduate from high school.

Is this insane?

I have an incredible talent for taking great news and turning it into an anxiety nightmare.

⌇

There are now these headaches.

Disabling ones.

I've had them on and off for about a year, but they've been getting worse in the summer of 2016, even since I got home from England. They are rendering me unable to do anything more than lie in bed, a sleep mask placed over my eyes as I listen to news on TV because looking at anything, never mind into the brightness of a screen, feels like someone's pulling my eyeballs out of my head as far as they can go without removing them. I stew in a rage because I'm trapped inside this flawed flesh vessel that's making it impossible for me to do anything other than lie here. I'm not reading. I'm not writing. I'm not walking the dogs. I'm not doing anything other than providing a warm, fleshy cushion for the thin, twelve-pound Tedy who likes to mash his black and tan body into my side (preferably between my legs or nestled into the small of my back), seeking warmth because I keep the house so cold.

Migraine-like episodes are happening with regularity. I see white, flashing spots which float in the periphery of my vision, as if I'm being partially blinded by fireflies. The bouts are frequently accompanied by a stabbing pain in the back, right-hand side of my head, where I sometimes experience a burning sensation as well. Nausea usually joins the party, as does that hungover feeling you get after having taken Nyquil or sleep medicine the night before, that head-is-disconnected-from-the-body feeling. For weeks at a time, I rise every morning with a crushing headache, having had not a drop of alcohol the night before.

I go to an optometrist. I get new eyeglasses—blue-black-rimmed progressive eyeglasses (the modern version of bifocals only without the telltale line across the bottom of the glass). The guy who helped me pick them out says they make me look very "writerly."

I inform Dr. Walker about these symptoms as I'm increasingly worried about what they mean. MS patients are urged to report any new symptoms to their neurologists because new symptoms may be indicative of an advancement of the disease.

"You need to get some more sleep," he tells me, adding that he'll prescribe me migraine and nausea medications. The migraine medication is incredibly effective at obliterating the mammoth pain. Sadly, I cannot regularly rely on it because Dr. Walker says it is addictive. Getting more sleep and using an over-the-counter migraine medicine are the best solutions he can offer. The anti-nausea medication helps when I experience migraine- and heat sensitivity-related nausea, works rapidly I discover. I begin carrying both of these prescription bottles in my purse everywhere I go, like a security blanket, as if they can protect me from the capricious nature of an unpredictable chronic disease.

⌐

Scott tells me I have been forgetting things.

I don't take this news well.

"I don't forget the *important* things!" I respond, defensively. "I remember what's going on *at work*. I don't forget what's going on in the news, or what I'm reading, or what I've seen!"

His declaration lightly touches the third rail of my worries.

Scott maintains a serene look before he closes his eyes and lowers his head. It's the face he makes when he's trying not to come across as patronizing, and because I know this, I gird myself to go on the defensive. He's silent for a moment or two, likely gathering his thoughts and choosing his words with tremendous care.

I fill that silence with wrath. "What? What have I forgotten? Were they things that mattered? Did I forget anything that mattered?" There's a raw vein of fear that's pulsating through my voice.

I don't want MS to go there. Not there.

He maintains his calm, resisting the urge to contemplatively stroke his salt-and-pepper goatee in that "The Thinker" posture he sometimes adopts but, in situations like this, makes me angry as I'm impulsive in discussions like this and don't want to wait for him to concoct his reasonable, patient, therapist-like response. I imagine he does this at work when delving into potentially volatile discussions. Here, with me, he is refraining from using his soft, I'm-so-much-calmer-than-you-are tone of voice that triggers me.

As we sit here at the kitchen table, I think about my mother and her forgetfulness. For years after Mom's first bout with cancer—breast cancer, which was beaten back by serious doses of near-lethal chemotherapy—her short-term memory became impaired, something she was loath to admit. She would forget whole conversations. She'd fail to recall that I told her I had plans on a given weekend and couldn't accompany her to a craft fair, then get angry because she had purchased tickets and was waiting for me at the entrance. She'd forget that we'd decided to have a Sunday family dinner at one p.m. instead of noon and chastise us for being late. When she was feeling charitable, she'd admit that she struggled with "chemo brain." But most of the time, she wasn't in a charitable mood. She was very, very proud, my mother.

"You haven't called in a month!" she would say on a Thursday evening.

"Mom, I talked to you on Sunday."

"No, you didn't."

"Yes, I did. I told you about Abbey's basketball game, the one where Scott argued with the refs. Remember?"

There would be a pause, the gears inside her brain would shift and adjust just enough to generate a vague recollection. Then there would be no sound from her end of the line.

"Do you remember that conversation?" I'd ask again, trying to tamp down my irritation, trying to remind myself that she wasn't intentionally being difficult.

At this point, Mom would change the subject. She would not say she was wrong. Apologies were for the weak. And I, a championship-level avoider of confrontation, would allow the conversational detour.

To attempt to avoid future arguments, I would make plans with her by email so she'd have a record to which she could refer, and to which I could refer (and aggressively email back to her to prove I was right) in the event of a misunderstanding. If we were making plans for a family gathering, for example, I'd copy Sean, my sister-in-law Lisa, and Scott on the email so everybody would be on the same page and no one could claim they weren't told anything.

After Mom died, I found her a series of leather-bound datebooks in her house. She always had one buried at the bottom of her gigantic, weighty purse that left red marks on her right shoulder. Despite having a smartphone, an iPad, and a laptop, Mom was very attached to her dead-tree datebooks. Leafing through the 2014 datebook years later, I discover that she used it as a tool to jog her memory, with notes from conversations and questions jotted down in the margins, alongside notations about what she did on any given day, with whom she spoke. Clearly, she knew she was having trouble but didn't want to concede any ground to anyone, lest she lose face.

Hmm.

I don't want to act like that, I realize as I settle onto a wooden kitchen chair. *I don't want to fight with Scott, to deny what may or may not be happening, no matter how much it may sting.*

"What have I been forgetting?" I ask quietly.

As gently as he can, he tells me that I have forgotten certain conversations I've had with him, like when we discussed that Jonah was going to be working at the ice cream shop on Sunday afternoon and that Casey had a hockey game at the same time. I forgot that Abbey was going to the movies with her friends that evening. I forgot that he had a meeting on a weeknight, even after he told me about it and inputted it into our shared digital calendar. My memory, I learn, has developed a sieve-like quality. Listening to Scott, I recognize I need to do something about this. Whether the something I need to do will make a difference in what appears to be happening is an open question.

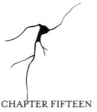

CHAPTER FIFTEEN

The Echo of His Touch

There's plenty of advice out there for spouses of people with MS. Multiple sclerosis websites offer bulletin boards and support groups, people on whom spouses can lean, people who get it. Alas, Scott's not a support group kind of guy. Sure, he *says* he looks at some of the links I email him, but he isn't really interested in doing a ton of research, or at least that's what he tells me.

Nearly two years since receiving my diagnosis, I continue to worry about the impact of this disease on my once 50-50, equitable marriage. I worry about feeling like the lesser partner, the one with the many, many needs. Scott may not say so, but I know he's concerned too. He's starting to talk about the types of places in which we'll live when we retire even though we're still in our forties. One-story living and accessibility frequently come up in these conversations, as do areas with colder climates. My takeaway: he's distressed about in what condition he thinks he may find me two decades from now. He's already envisioning me in worst case scenario condition.

In the meantime, I make another appointment with Dr. Walker to see him in November 2016. My next scheduled appointment wasn't until February 2017. But I need to see the doctor sooner. Although the combination of getting more sleep and taking the new medicine Dr. Walker prescribed has helped me cope with my headaches, I'm experiencing new symptoms that are wearing away at my soul and adding new wrinkles to Scott's forehead. And I'm not just talking about the memory issues Scott has identified.

⌐

I am lying on my right side, facing toward the two windows in my bedroom on a beautiful fall 2016 evening. Both windows are open, and I can feel the fresh air on my face. I need sleep. Gobs and gobs of it. I want to inhale sleep. Mainline it. Absorb as much sleep as I possible. It's as if I can never get enough to fill the sleep-deficit I have. The new semester is in full swing both at the university where I teach journalism—where we're now focused on news coverage of the general presidential election—and with my MFA classes where I'm deep into working on my thesis.

Scott wants to make me feel good, wants to soothe me. In the dark, I feel his hand on my back, rubbing deeply into my shoulders, into my shoulder blades, the back of my neck. I had been complaining about lugging my laptop and other heavy items around campus and he is trying to address the aches. He can't pierce my flesh and my bones and delve into my brain or into my spinal cord to extract the lesions that are fouling up his wife's health. But relieving shoulder aches? That he can do. His massage gets more intense as he tries to loosen up the knots, to loosen me up after, what was for me, a long day that left me spent, or, as my son Casey likes to say, left me gassed.

It's at this moment when I become acutely aware of the changes in my body. As his hands alternatively dig deep into muscles and skim over my skin, I notice the sensation of his fingertips on sections of my flesh are dramatically diminished. While I have been experiencing reduced-sensitivity on both of my legs recently—particularly on the top of my feet, and on top of my hands—under cover of the darkness I become acutely aware that larger territories are being overtaken, swallowed up by encroaching numbness. My back. My abdomen. My chest. It's as though an application of Novocain that had been injected into my epidermis is in the middle stages of wearing off. It's so strange. Your clothes wear strangely against your skin, like your skin is not entirely your own. Someone else's touch seems far away.

Scott continues the massage unaware that his touch has triggered an altogether different reaction inside of me than what he's aiming for: dread not romance. The massaging, while meant to be nurturing and loving, suddenly reminds me, *all is not normal here*. My skin is sending off-kilter messages to my brain, indicating that something's awry. In my lower belly, it slightly stings as his hand draws across it. I know there's nothing on my belly, no cuts, no wounds, no rashes, no irritating bug bites. The stinging is just a byproduct of MS-ravaged nerves. Nonsense messages being ferried between my brain and spinal cord to the rest of my body are responsible for the stinging sensation.

I close my eyes and try to consciously force myself to relax, to deeply appreciate this nice thing my husband is trying to do for me. But my mind keeps returning to the new way the touch of skin to skin feels on my body. It doesn't feel like a touch, more like an echo of a touch, an echo that I dread will eventually fade as the last note disappears in the air. Instead of enjoying it, I'm mourning the way I used to feel, the woman I once was.

⌒

Before I visit Dr. Walker, I sit at my desk and pull out the blue and tan notebook into which I've been documenting my symptoms. It's a motley collection. Headaches. Numbness. Fatigue. Periodic eye issues with sparkly spots in my peripheral vision.

New on the list is altered taste:

Nothing tastes "normal" anymore. I sit down in the sun-room one Sunday afternoon with a box of Ritz crackers at my side and the day's newspapers on my lap when I pop a whole cracker into my mouth, salt-side down. I want to relish the salty grains, as I'm a savory snacks kinda person. Only problem is, I can't feel the grains on my tongue. Thinking that maybe it's just something wacky with a single cracker, I try another one. Same thing. Over the next several days, I test myself to see if it is just a one-off experience. I later discover that my hazelnut coffee tastes burnt. The Italian wine Scott and I love—Cantina Zaccagnini (we refer to it as the "stick wine" because it comes with a twig fastened to the bottle)—tastes acidic and sour in my mouth, but tastes great to Scott. The after-dinner drink we sip occasionally, Grand Marnier, a cognac blended with orange, seems rubbing alcohol harsh to me, but com-pletely normal to Scott. Marinara sauce, even well spiced, seems bland, but then I notice the kids are fanning their mouths at the dinner table because they tell me it's extremely spicy. Nearly everything I eat or drink does not taste the way I think it should. I do not have a cold. My nose is not stuffed up.

As I am wont to do, I take to my laptop seeking to learn if this sudden alteration to my taste is potentially related to MS.

"It's probably one of the lesser-reported symptoms of MS, but a research team at the University of Pennsylvania's Smell and Taste Center concluded that there is a high incidence of poor ability to identify taste by people with MS," an English website, Overcoming Multiple Sclerosis, says about a *Journal of Neurology* study. "Little had previously been known or stud-ied regarding the relationship between taste and MS, although former research estimated that between 5 to 20 percent of people with MS experienced some kind of taste dysfunction."

I find a couple of other pieces referring to that same *Journal of Neurology* study, then discover an intriguing blog post on the Everyday Health website from 2006 written by a classically trained chef with MS who loses his sense of taste, particularly of salty items. "A big 'hole' appeared in the center of my tongue, where salt receptors are concentrated," the man writes. "I wasn't tasting salt. ... Toothpaste was shockingly sweet, pasta tastes like its namesake—paste, coffee is nothing but aftertaste."

Taste is off, I write in my notebook which I plan to bring to my upcoming appointment with Dr. Walker.

I mentally comb through recent weeks trying to remember experiences that are atypical for me, experiences that may or may not be related to the MS. My mind goes to my commute to the university one recent afternoon. While driving the twenty-five miles from my house to Boston on the Massachusetts Turnpike, I experience spasms across the top of my right ankle when I pressed the gas pedal. The spasms last only a couple of seconds. It is more irritating and surprising than painful. When it occurs, it is hard to think about anything other than my ankle, but since I am driving, I should really be paying attention to the road.

This is weird, I think.

Then it happens again. Then a few times more. When I get to school, it recedes, which is fortunate, given that I am wearing high-heeled shoes and really don't want to take a stumble because of an ankle spasm while in front of my undergraduates. A more severe, stabbing-pain version of this right ankle spasm resurfaces numerous times over the next few weeks, mostly when I am lying in bed trying to go to sleep or sitting still for an extended period of time. For a few consecutive evenings, it is so aggravating that it interrupts my sleep. I stretch my legs out, flex, and shake them to try to relax the muscles. I get out of bed, put my hands on the edge of the mattress, and do some leg stretches in the dark, trying to avoid accidentally stepping on Max who likes to sleep on the floor next to the bed. None of this puts an end to the spasms. Worried I am disturbing Scott, I give up on sleeping in our shared bed, go downstairs, turn on the gas fireplace, read a book, and rotate my ankles, knowing I will pay for my sleeplessness the following day with headaches and a foggy brain. The National Multiple Sclerosis Society's website I consult the next day tells me spasticity "is one of the more common symptoms of MS." *Ankle and legs spasms, sleep problems* goes into my notebook of symptoms.

Lest I forget, as I document my latest symptoms on a list of things about which to ask the neurologist, I must add difficulties concentrating. Over the past months, I have been experiencing difficulties reading newspapers. My three newspapers are reliable friends who greet me every day and thrill me with new and interesting stories and ideas. I adore reading the hard copies because I'm really into the whole tactile experience of it, ink-stained fingers be damned. This routine is not all that far removed from what I watched my father do when I was a kid. Although he didn't drink coffee—Mom was the java addict—he would flip on NBC's *Today Show* in the mornings before work while he read the local newspaper. Mom hated how he left newspapers lying around (much like Scott's reaction when he finds articles I jaggedly ripped from pages and left in various places). Dad's parents before him were heavy newspaper readers and TV news watchers. This is a routine that seems preordained. It gets me ready for my day. It makes me feel ready to write, to teach journalism, to be an involved, knowledgeable citizen of the world. When I miss this coffee-and-papers routine (even though coffee isn't tasting quite right to me lately), the day never seems right. And now, my favorite part of the day appears to be in jeopardy.

Here's what's been happening: I will start to read an article, like the lead story in the *New York Times*, which is typically about a serious topic. I will read down to the third paragraph, my vision will blur a little (despite my new glasses), and I'll forget what I just read. The context of the third paragraph will make no sense. So, I go back to the beginning. Then it happens again.

Maybe I'm just bored with this story or don't like how it's written.

This happens again and again, mostly on mornings when I haven't had a lot of quality sleep the previous night. I switch newspapers. I pick up *The Boston Globe*. Same thing.

What the hell is happening? I ask myself.

I push the papers aside and instead listen to CNN morning hosts on the TV. I'm easily able to understand the news when I hear them discuss it. The reading part has become—on many mornings—a challenge lately. It's not an omnipresent challenge but it happens frequently enough that it makes me feel distinctly uncomfortable.

A formerly boastful multitasker, who used to pride myself on reading and writing quickly and with brutal efficiency in noisy newsrooms, my mental focus is now easily obliterated by shiny and noisy objects. When I become frustrated that I cannot read through a news story, it's easier to focus on Tedy, who's dragging an eviscerated stuffed cow across the kitchen floor, and to engage him in two dozen rounds of fetch. As my irritation about my inability to focus escalates, I find myself looking up from my reading material seeking any escape route disguised as an urgent chore. If a *Globe* op/ed is giving me trouble, I'll look up and notice the collection of seltzer cans on the kitchen counter that needs to be recycled.

Well I can do that, bring them to the recycling bin, I think. It makes me feel better, more in charge, to collect those cans and deposit them in the bin in the garage and listen to the satisfying sound of cans hitting other cans instead of struggling with the morass of words that is vexing me because a snafu involving damaged nerves in my brain is temporarily prohibiting me from reading properly.

The periodic struggles I'm having with the written word encompass more than simply reading the newspapers. Grading my students' news analyses about the newspaper front pages during the tumultuous 2016 presidential campaign should be catnip for me, a news hound who is obsessed with politics. But it's proving to be a long, agonizing slog. I will start reading a student's submission, re-read the first paragraph a few times, then wrestle with my brain to stay on task, forbidding myself to check Twitter or email. I'm acting as though I have an attention deficit disorder problem. And, in a way, I do. One part of my brain is telling me to do something else other than what I'm doing, my conscious mind is shouting, *Get to work! Read this paper!* Without realizing it, I'm bribing myself to push through the difficulties and get through one paper. *If you finish this paper, THEN you can check Twitter.* Or *You can get yourself another can of seltzer when you've graded three assignments.* I am antsy. I cannot get my brain to settle down. It feels like I'm going mad.

If I cannot read and cannot focus, how can I succeed as a writer and as an educator? Is this MS or is this just aging or fatigue?

I write *difficulty concentrating* on my list of ailments.

Armed with my list, I head into Boston to see Dr. Walker in early November 2016 hoping for some information and, possibly, solutions.

What I don't do is more closely examine my MRI reports, the ones that indicate a lesion in the middle section of my corpus callosum, the area which governs communication between the left and right hemispheres of the brain. Much later, Dr. Walker will tell me this "might slow down your ability to process things."

‿

I leave Dr. Walker's office feeling foolish. The fortysomething bespectacled doctor with the salt-and-pepper goatee responds to the altered taste symptom I report to him with a quick, "I've never heard of that before." Because my complaint largely involves lack of sensation and taste in the middle of my tongue, he says that's not a concern because any anomalies related to MS would have to involve the whole tongue. (A few years later, he takes my complaints about a loss of taste more seriously and informs me he's heard from other patients who have the same experience. Alas, Dr. Walker said, there's no treatment options available to restore my taste sensations.)

On the matter of my challenges concentrating, Dr. Walker initially suggests I take ADHD medication, another prescription I'd have to take every day. For the rest of my life. The case he makes for this medicine doesn't persuade me enough to fill the prescription. And I tell him so. I'm already taking a lot of stuff, and I don't want to add another, permanent medication to my regimen. Not yet.

He accepts my rejection matter-of-factly but suggests that it's a good idea for me to be evaluated by the hospital's cognitive neurology team in order to establish a baseline measure for my memory, concentration, and cognition. Getting an evaluation will provide an assessment of where I am now so should anything change, we can measure that change. I know how important quantifiable measurements are to Dr. Walker. He's a huge fan of data. He seems to worship it above all else. Numbers are reliable, patients, not so much. I agree to submit myself to such an examination, which will take place on the day before Scott and I host Thanksgiving.

My report about the intermittent spasms in my right ankle yields a recommendation from Dr. Walker that I take an over-the-counter medication with magnesium specifically meant to combat nighttime leg cramps. He gives me prescription for a muscle relaxant.

I tell him more areas of my body are losing sensation. I detail which areas and offer him an anecdote from the previous week: I am working on my laptop, grading a student's paper online while sitting at the kitchen table. In the middle of grading, I decide to take a break and take out the recycling that is on the kitchen counter. I carry several plastic bottles and one empty can of dog food out to the garage. When I return to my laptop, I resume typing. A short time later, I look down and see blood smeared over the left-hand side of the keyboard.

What the hell? I blurt. Blood has dripped onto the placemat and my lap. As I rinse off my left hand in cold water, I spot the cut on my left pinky finger, obviously from the jagged edge of the can of dog food. The strange thing is, as the water runs down and into the cut, I feel nothing. No stinging. Normally, I would feel the sting as well as the wetness of the blood on my hand.

Dr. Walker sits still for a moment. He cocks his head to the side. The pause is long. He is thinking. Then he says, "Well, I sometimes cut my hand and don't notice it."

I say nothing.

There's another pause.

He moves on.

Maybe it really isn't a big deal, I think. *Maybe* everything *isn't MS-related.* It's hard for me, a layperson to tell. How am I supposed to know what's normal and what isn't? For someone whose first MS symptom was numbness, whose complaints of numbness were initially dismissed as likely the result of anxiety, I think this is possibly significant. But, as I said, I'm not a neurologist.

During another exchange following my physical exam, whose results mirror the ones from several months before, Dr. Walker admits he likes things that can be objectively measured. Like this peg-in-a-hole test he has me do to assess hand-eye coordination. He sets the timer on his iPhone and has me use my right hand to pick up plastic pegs from a round well next to a plastic board and, one by one, place the pegs in the holes in the board as fast as I can, followed by removing them, individually, and returning them to the well. Then I repeat the task with the left hand. What Dr. Walker likes about the peg test is the crisp surety of it. It yields times he can measure against previous and future scores. He can examine the results and determine if my manual dexterity is diminishing or stable. Patient-reported symptoms—like explaining diminished sensation across my body, that "my coffee tastes like it's burned" and "my red wine tastes too acidic"—cannot be measured by the clinician. These symptoms are thoroughly subjective. They are claims made by me, the fallible patient.

During a later discussion about MS symptoms like lightheadedness, Dr. Walker says, "[D]izziness or other squirrely symptoms are squishy and subjective. Forget what [the patient] says. What does the MRI say?"

Physicians, from my experience, tend to assess the veracity of their patients (which is, ironically, also a subjective measure) in order to determine if the new symptoms they report are serious. Stories about unmeasurable symptoms are not clean like data and lab reports. But many MS symptoms, like fatigue and nausea, are unquantifiable, impossible to be measured by an external, unbiased machine, and, therefore, are easily dismissed since there is no one test that can say, "Yessirree! This patient is more fatigued than someone of her age and level of fitness should be. So says the blood test." Or, "This report says her level of taste is significantly altered, seventy-five percent differentiation from her normal taste sensations."

With each shrug and benign utterance of, "I've never heard of that," I feel like that uncertain little girl I once was, someone who frets about being told she doesn't know anything. These non-reactions make me reluctant to talk about any "new" symptoms I may experience for fear I'll wind up feeling stupid like I did when Dr. Sabine explained away my numbness as "psychosomatic." If I ever experience some of the more intimate and embarrassing symptoms of MS—sexual dysfunction, loss of bladder or bowel control—I will be reticent to muster the courage to mention them because I don't want them inadvertently dismissed as unrelated or irrelevant, even if they're dismissed in Dr. Walker's polite and quiet fashion.

Later, I read Dr. Walker's medical notes to see what he writes about this visit:

She notes increased headaches, and lack of sleep. She thinks Fioricet [the migraine medication] is partly beneficial. She notes some cognitive focus issues but does not think headaches are a factor. She has a class of 50 students and has trouble getting through the papers. She also notes some decreased sensation and taste in middle of tongue. She cut her finger on the left hand without feeling this once recently. She also has some R foot numbness over the last few weeks. She also notes some nausea and whoozy [sic] feeling recently. Zofran helps nausea (for the last 2 weeks has been more frequent). Whooziness [sic] has been infrequent but did take one day off school, staying in bed. She can also get leg cramps overnight.

Okay, I think, *he got most of what I was saying and didn't pass judgment, at least not in the official record. That's encouraging.*

Dr. Walker outlines the plan: keep taking the medicine he has prescribed for the headaches and nausea, take Vitamin D, get another MRI, get my every-six-month blood tests, take magnesium meds as needed for spasms, get more quality sleep, and consider a trial prescription of a potent medicine for headaches (the only thing which I decline).

The following week, I receive mixed signals about my latest MRI and a seemingly contradictory desires bloom inside me: I want the MRI to provide evidence of new or inflamed lesions to give my evidence-seeking neurologist something tangible to explain my new and worsening symptoms, although, at the same time, I *don't* want the MRI results to indicate advancement of the disease. Without MRI evidence, I worry about Dr. Walker's response to my reports of unquantifiable symptoms. I want to have proof that I'm not insane. This desire makes no sense, intellectually. I don't want my disease to progress. I don't want new lesions. What I want is validation. I remain very sensitive to the very hint from a physician that I'm fabricating or, perhaps if I want to be more generous, that I'm exaggerating what I'm experiencing.

Around this same time, I start researching how female patients are treated by the medical world. The research is damning. Having a physician question a female patient's story, questioning her reporting what's going on in her own body, is, unfortunately, not unusual. It is quite prevalent, this notion of "female pain" being "perceived as constructed or exaggerated," as writer Leslie Jamison says. In an October 2015 *Atlantic* piece, "How Doctors Take Women's Pain Less Seriously," writer Joe Fassler chronicles his wife's emergency room experience when nurses and doctors doubt her reports of excruciating abdominal pain. What she was experiencing was something called "ovarian torsion," a twisted ovary, which a medical journal calls "a true surgical emergency," Fassler writes. However, the medical staffers at the hospital don't believe that his wife Rachel needs immediate attention and treat her writhing pain with indifferent contempt, labeling her as non-emergent. After hours of waiting and being snapped at by disbelieving medical personnel, Fassler says a doctor finally examines the results of a CT scan and discovers his wife has "a large mass in her abdomen." There's the objective, scientific report that many physicians require, because, you know, you can't take a female patient's word for it.

Fassler's piece leads me to the 2001 *The Journal of Law, Medicine & Ethics'* article "The Girl Who Cried Pain: A Bias Against Women in the Treatment of Pain" by Professors Diane E. Hoffmann and Anita J. Tarzian, which found that women's pain is undertreated and met with great skepticism by medical professionals. "The subjective nature of pain requires health care providers to view the patient as a credible reporter, and stereotypes or assumptions about behavior in such circumstances (oversensitivity, complaining, stoicism) add to the likelihood of under-treatment of some groups and over-treatment of others," the report says. "... Physicians have found women to have more 'psychosomatic illnesses, more emotional lability and more complaints due to emotional factors' than men."

When it comes to female patients, it seems, the medical folks want the cold, hard facts. "In Western medicine, health-care providers are trained to rely predominantly on objective evidence of disease and injury," Hoffmann and Tarzian write. "… The medical model overemphasizes objective, biological indicators of pain and under-acknowledges women's subjective, experiential reports."

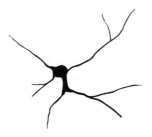

CHAPTER SIXTEEN
Adventures in Cognitive Neurology

MS has the potential to affect mood, personality and cognition—
the attributes that make us unique—either directly or indirectly. The
idea is upsetting, but the facts emerging from research are encourag-
ing—while mild to moderate problems are relatively common, severe
damage to these aspects of the self are not.

  – National Multiple Sclerosis Society's "Managing Cognitive
    Problems in MS"

"Which cognitive functions might be affected by MS?" asks
the National Multiple Sclerosis Society?
The group's website answers its own question:
• Memory and/or recall
• Attention and concentration
• Speed of information processing
• Abstract reasoning, problem-solving and executive
  functions
• Visual-spatial abilities
• Verbal fluency
"...[W]hile the majority of people with MS will experience
cognitive changes, the changes for most will be mild to mod-
erate," the Society says.
Other than offering methods to cope with these changes,
the Society says there's no single, iron-clad way of stopping
them.

On exercise: "There has been increasing interest in the potential of physical exercise to improve cognitive function both in healthy adults and individuals with chronic conditions such as Alzheimer's and MS."

On medications: "At present, the pharmacy has little to offer; research clearly needs to continue."

⌇

I have no rational explanation for why I cannot see the vacuum cleaner I need in order to clean up debris left in the family room after our hounds, Max and Tedy, raid the pantry and tear into a box of hot chocolate packets. True, I am in a rush. I am nearly ready to leave the house to go to teach at the university when I notice that Max, who I recently put on a diet because he has started to become rounder than he should be, and yappy little Tedy, have ripped open hot cocoa packets they nicked from our pantry. The voracious consumption of the pilfered packets leaves tan saliva-covered circles all over the off-white rug in the family room. I rush around the house looking for the vacuum cleaner. Okay, so maybe I'm not *really* looking, not in earnest anyway. That's the only reason I can think of to explain why I do not see the vacuum cleaner in the middle of Scott's office closet, the one Scott locates with ease later that night.

For me, this is a disturbing role reversal. During the many years in which we've been a couple, Scott has been the one who cannot find things. He's the one who will be searching in vain for the ketchup in the fridge, only to have me swoop in and sarcastically point out that the bottle is in front of his face. I am the item-finder. I am the one who always knows where everything is.

"I don't think we have any more pasta," he would say, emerging from the pantry.

"Yes, we do."

"No, I just looked."

Arching my left eyebrow, "Do I need to go over there and find it? I *know* it's there."

"We don't have any."

I walk over, grab the box of pasta that's roughly eye-level, smirk, and hand it to him, debating whether an "I told you so" is too over-the-top, or whether it needs to be said at all. Nine times-out-of-ten, any time Scott is looking for a household item while trapped in his personal cocoon of item-blindness, I find the item in question. The fact that I did not see the vacuum cleaner that was in full view and in its normal place, unmoors me.

Later that evening, after the hot chocolate packet canine massacre, Scott goes to his office and re-appears in the kitchen. He has the vacuum in his hands. He looks worried. "It was right there. In the middle, front of the closet. You couldn't miss it," he says. His brow furrows, something that's happening more often these days.

A couple weeks later, Jonah needs help finding a shiny, metal bin into which we put bottles of beverages and cover with ice when we're hosting a large event. Together, my item-blind son and I search the garage and Scott's office, including the closets. We turn up nothing and report our failure to Scott who, upon hearing this, closes his eyes and looks at the floor. He disappears and quickly re-emerges from the basement with the bin.

"Where the hell did you find that?" I ask, incredulous.

"In the closet in my office."

Usually, proving me wrong, particularly wrong when it comes to locating a lost item, would fill Scott with glee. Not so today.

I stand in the kitchen, stunned, just as I had been with the vacuum cleaner. "In the closet? But I checked the closet. I looked. Really."

What is it with me and that damned closet?

"It was behind the gift bags."

Did I check under the gift bags? Did I look for the hint of shiny metal? The fact that I cannot recall if I checked under or behind the gift bags, that I am unsure about how I conducted my search, fills me with dread. *Did I not see it? Was I not concentrating? What the hell?* Throw in Scott's recently-voiced concerns that I'm becoming forgetful about minor things, and that I'm having trouble concentrating when I read the newspaper and grade papers, and couple it with the fact that Dr. Walker has suggested that I undergo a cognitive neurological exam, and it's collectively enough to take my legs out from under me.

Am I losing my mind?

I am a writer. It's who I am. I require proper cognitive functioning in order to do this. While some cling to other roles in their lives—like being a wife, mother, daughter, and sister, all roles I deeply cherish—in my DNA, I love words, I love putting them together, shaping them into something meaningful. But somewhere in my programming, there's malware, a malicious piece of code that queued my immune system to assault nerves in my brain and spinal cord, and it now threatens my very core.

⤸

The cognitive neurology unit personnel at the hospital are very attentive during my day-before-Thankgiving 2016 consultation. They watch everything I do and say, in a slightly creepy, Big Brother-ish kind of way. In their clinical notes I obtain after my visit, they include their assessment of me:

She arrived 30 minutes early for her appointment. She was well groomed and appropriately attired. She was cooperative, socially engaging, dynamic and personable. She was alert and fully oriented (date, day, month, year, state, city, county and hospital) and was aware of topical events. During the testing, she approached all tasks with enthusiasm although she expressed dismay with tasks that involved numbers due to lifelong weakness with mathematics. She appeared anxious initially; however, anxiety subsided as testing progressed. On a word recognition task, she stumbled on a number of high-frequency words, but was able to correctly pronounce words after a few attempts. Thought processes were logical and linear. Thought content was congruent with the topics discussed. Mood was rated as four to five out of a maximum of 10. She described herself feeling apprehensive.

Having one's mental faculties assessed is akin to being naked in a room full of clothed people who are scrutinizing every bulge, every fold, and every blemish on your body. Being shown a dizzying array of geometric shapes and asked which one comes next in the series, being asked to name the animals depicted in drawings, to literally connect the dots alternating between ascending numbers and letters, to recite a list of non-sequential numbers backwards, to draw an analog clock, to copy a cube drawing, to remember a bizarre sketch and recreate it several minutes later from memory with colored pencils under a time constraint, and to recall a list of unrelated words long after they are first introduced to you, all while knowing you're being watched and that the results being recorded and inputted into your medical records, makes you feel like a skittish lab rat. And I am feeling very rat-like this morning.

At one point during the exam, I am asked to name "all the words that start with the letter F." When the young neurologist with the long, dark hair, and intense gaze gives me this directive (she is, quite possibly, a resident in training), I start to quietly panic.

I don't actually know every word that starts with the letter F. Is she being literal? That can't be, right. Nobody knows ALL the words. The gigantic Oxford English Dictionary with its thousands of pages pops into my head. While I have this debate inside my head about the possibility of anyone knowing every word that starts with F, the timer on her smartphone is ticking away and I'm losing precious moments in which I can start uttering words that start with an F. Every second that elapses without me naming one of those words is another strike against me, against my mental abilities. I try to shake myself out of this mental tangent and focus on her question.

Focus damn it! I shout inside my head, hoping the woman can't tell that I'm freaking out. You start feeling paranoid when you're sitting inside the stuffy, darkened womb-like room facing the door with its tiny window, a window is like ... *Stop it!* I tell myself as I think about what the room looks like. *Stop creating similes!*

The testing goes on for what seems like a very long time. About fifteen minutes into it, I'm starting to sweat, from both nervousness and the fact that the room is overheated, and I'm worried I'll suffer an MS exacerbation. I ask the young examiner if she can turn off the heater. She obliges. Distracted by so many things right now, the heat doesn't have to be one of them.

The cognitive neurologist in charge, Dr. O'Leary, makes an appearance in the small exam room which already feels crowded with two people inside. To me, she looks like she's in her late fifties or early sixties. Her blond-gray bob sways gently as speaks with a voice that's touched by a bit of bronchitis. Amid her warbly small talk, she asks some questions about my background, my education, my work. Dr. O'Leary departs shortly after this, leaving the testing to her protégé.

The tests, I later learn, have an array of names: the Montreal Cognitive Assessment (MoCA) which screens for mild cognitive impairment, the Wechsler Adult Intelligence Scale (WAIS) which measures intelligence, the Conners Continuous

Performance Test that gauges inattentiveness and impulsivity, the Boston Naming Test that assesses word retrieval for the brain-damaged, the California Verbal Learning Test which evaluates verbal recall, the Rey Complex Figure Test which examines a multitude of abilities ranging from working memory to planning, and the Matrix Reasoning Test that appraises patients' visual-spatial problem solving.

How do I fare during my high-stakes testing? Days later, I receive an email from Dr. O'Leary's office telling me my results are available online. While I have an appointment slated for the following week, the first week of December 2016, to discuss the results in person, I am compelled to immediately read the results online. I need to know where I stand. I'm home alone in my office, so if I have an emotional reaction, only the cocoa-packet-eating dogs will be there to witness it. I'll be safe from being embarrassed by my reaction to any bad news. And it's that bad news I fear, that my mental abilities are being hampered by a disease with no cure, that things will go nothing but downhill from here on out. I really don't want to read these results, but I know I must.

"[O]verall premorbid intellectual capacity was estimated to fall in the high average to superior range. [O'Brien's] scores on tests sampling various neurocognitive domains were interpreted in consideration of this benchmark," the report says.

Tests on which I do relatively well: short-term auditory attention, processing visual information, retrieving the name of pictured objects, semantic fluency, learning and remembering a list of words, and verbal recognition memory. Troublesome areas include a sustained attention test. "Testing was notable for a reduction in response speed in later blocks ... suggesting some difficulties with sustained attention. ... Testing was notable for some problems with maintaining vigilance."

This, I think, *makes me sound like a negligent superhero not maintaining my vigilance over Gotham, like I somehow missing the Bat Signal because I was napping.*

The report's conclusion:

The functional impact of these test findings is that [O'Brien] may encounter difficulties transiently holding, processing and manipulating information subsumed by variable working memory performance. She may struggle with multitasking and regulating concentration for long periods of time. Regarding memory, her working memory weakness will impact her ability to digest and simultaneously process a large volume of verbal information initially; however, she can circumvent this weakness when provided with repetition. Testing suggests she still may encounter difficulties spontaneously retrieving information from memory when under time constraints; however, with practice and extra time she will be able to compensate. Overall, the neuropsychological profile is notable for subtle cognitive decline, preferentially involving some aspects of executive system functioning consistent with the cognitive sequelae associated with multiple sclerosis.

∽

Dad doesn't show up for Thanksgiving dinner at my house. He says he's sick. Only, as I'm working on preparing the festive dishes for my family of five plus my Dad, I don't know that he has decided not to come.

Jonah and Casey are riveted by their video games in the basement. Scott and I are divvying up the recipe cards and working in the kitchen as Abbey watches the Thanksgiving Day parade on TV, joining us after Santa goes by. We prepare several family favorites which we hope will please Dad, like the corn casserole dish, whose recipe Mom got from someone at the annual Strawberry Supper at our old church, the same church where my parents were married months before I was born. Abbey makes a homemade apple pie with which we will serve slices of sharp Vermont cheddar cheese alongside the slices, just as Dad likes it. The kitchen is brimming with swirling aromas of the roast turkey, the corn bread and mushroom stuffing, the butternut squash puree with the pecan and brown sugar topping, and the savory mashed potatoes, heavy with salt and fresh rosemary and chicken broth. I'm humming along to the upbeat music I'm playing from my phone—some Stevie Wonder, some U2—genuinely happy, as I finish my part of the food prep and head upstairs to shower and get dressed.

After one o'clock comes and goes and Dad has yet to arrive, I start to get worried. It takes about an hour-and-a-half to drive from his house to mine, without traffic. By one-thirty, I call his cell phone to find out where he is. It goes directly to voicemail, a message Abbey recorded for him years ago. I don't leave a message because he says he doesn't know (and is unwilling to learn) how to retrieve his voicemail messages. I call his land line at his house which is answered by the machine and a recording of my mother's voice, a recording which never fails to make me flinch every time I hear it. He doesn't pick up the house phone. I call again. And again.

My imagination spits out images for me to consider: Dad in a car accident and he's unconscious. Dad's car has gone off the side of the road and he's unable to reach his cell phone. Dad has fallen in the house and cannot get up off the floor to reach a phone. Any wistfulness I was enjoying during the morning is replaced by anxiousness, the calm replaced by a stomach-ache.

By two o'clock, Dad finally calls my house. He's hoarse and coughing loudly directly into the receiver.

"I called you" hack, hack, aggressive clearing of the throat "this morning an left you a message telling you I was sick."

"I never got that message. I've been cooking all morning. Are you okay?"

"I've got this cold and I'm in bed. I'll be fine but I need to go back to bed."

"Why didn't you pick up your cell or your house phone when I called all those times?"

"I was sleeping."

When the call ends, I go to my office where my answering machine resides in my office, to see if he left a message.

While I'm walking, I consider how I could have missed *his* call. The door to my office is usually kept closed so the resident hounds won't get into trouble in there and do something stupid like overturning the waste basket and rummage through the trash. And if you consider that everybody who lives in this house tends to leave the many handsets for the land line all over the place—under comforters in their beds, between sofa cushions, in the basement next to the Xbox, or just languishing on the bedroom floor where the charge has run out—it's no wonder no one heard the phone when it rang at nine o'clock in the morning. The message light is indeed blinking red. I listen to his message. He was telling the truth. My relief that he is not dead and has not been in a motor vehicle accident and is not lying on the floor in his house, injured and shouting into the void is rapidly supplanted by disappointment.

I text my brother to vent. Turns out, Sean already knew Dad wasn't coming to Thanksgiving dinner at my house. He knew about it *yesterday* when Dad informed him was too ill to join us for dinner, and then go to Sean's house for dessert. I share my extreme disappointment with my brother, and we commiserate. Dad has repeatedly cancelled plans on both my family and Sean's during the past two years. He typically calls whoever extends the invitation at the last minute and tell us that 1) he is sick 2) his dog Kelly is sick 3) his car is dead (the automotive version of being sick), or 4) that Kelly is so old that he might die while Dad is at our house and he doesn't want to risk leaving him home alone.

While I speak with Dad during our weekly calls—he talks more often with Sean—the details he shares of his daily life indicate he has retreated into his own, insular world. It's not that he's not getting out of the house; he is. Kind of. He has his friends at the local pub he frequents, where he now has a regular seat on the far corner of the bar. He sees his brother once a week, oftentimes going out to lunch together and then going to the local Barnes & Noble, or they get together for dinner at my uncle and his wife's house. Dad gets his take-out on regular basis from his regular places, including the Italian family restaurant at the end of the street. And he is on Facebook, mostly either liking or disliking stuff, and sharing things like announcements about lost dogs and political memes.

But neither Sean nor I see him in person very often. Despite our repeated entreaties for him to witness our children's life events (their school concerts and award ceremonies, their Little League games and track and field events), to celebrate holidays with us, or to simply break bread with one another, more often than not, it doesn't happen. He's has told us he doesn't like to drive on the Turnpike, so we've offered to have him stay over at one of our houses, so he wouldn't have to take the highway twice on the same day. He doesn't take us up on those offers. We now go months and months without seeing him. When we visit him at his house, it feels like he wants us to leave as soon as possible, like he's no longer comfortable with having us in his space. The conversations we have with the guy who, five years earlier, could have given master classes in small talk, are sadly stilted.

I'm left to speculate about what's happening. Perhaps he doesn't like it when Sean or I try to tidy the kitchen. Maybe it feels invasive when we suggest that we remove the clean clothing from completely covering the sofa or that we remove the mail that's piled on the kitchen chairs so there will be a place for us to sit. When there's no place for you to sit down when you're visiting someone, it doesn't feel as though your presence is desired.

Once I saw an empty pill pack lying on the kitchen counter

and was about to throw it out, when he said, "Leave it! Leave it!"

"But Dad, it's from two years ago. Why is it out here? Shouldn't you just throw it out?"

"No, just leave it!"

During one visit, my sister-in-law was about to throw out a dead, moldy houseplant and Dad admonished her not to move it. The plant must've been purchased by Mom—Dad never would've purchased a plant—but now it was shriveled up and smelled. It needed to go. But Dad wanted it to remain in place.

I can only try to imagine what this is like for him, to be living in the house, surrounded by my mother's things, frozen in time, unwilling to plunge forward into a new, terrible reality, into a retirement that is the polar opposite of what he thought it would be. I'm sure he hates having Sean or me come into his house and point out that there are dead plants and empty pill packs lying around that need to go into the garbage. I'm sure he hates feeling as though he's being judged for the state of his home. I'm sure he aches for things to be the way they used to be, with easy conversations, delicious homemade food, and warmth inside that kitchen, filled with people and laughter. That would explain why he sometimes calls us a few hours before we're supposed to drive out to see him and tells us not to come. The reasons for the cancellations vary.

It's as though our relationship with him withered, like that houseplant, and is sitting in the windowsill, dying from neglect. I don't know what to do about it. I am heartsick.

Both Sean and I have offered to have holiday dinners at his house, to prepare and bring the food, but Dad doesn't embrace those suggestions. When they're tossed out there, he doesn't bite. He seems content to have a telephonic relationship. Without my mother, he seems as though he can't bear to gather together with family, like it's somehow wrong. Instead, he's removed himself from the picture as well, so when my family and Sean's family get together for holidays, there are two empty seats at the table which consume more emotional room than any one person who's actually sitting there.

After I tell the kids that Grandpa isn't coming to our 2016 Thanksgiving meal, Abbey—who lovingly prepared many of the dishes and who has acutely misses her grandmother's presence—weeps.

〜

The week after Thanksgiving, I return to the overheated, tastefully-appointed Cognitive Neurology waiting room, with its colorful abstract images and large painting on the back wall with an ocean-blue strip across the top half of the canvas and a black strip across the bottom, reminding me of something Mark Rothko might have created. As I settle into my waiting room seat and check email messages, I wonder whether I'm being watched, whether my arrival time and attire have already been noted. In short order, I'm summoned to Dr. O'Leary's office.

Not trusting myself to remember the details of the conversation, I pull out my iPhone, place it on the table in front of me, and ask Dr. O'Leary if she minds if I record our session. She says she does not mind and, after giving her consent, plunges right into summarizing the tests which she says attempt to measure patients' "premorbid abilities."

"That 'premorbid' sounds terrible," I say as I emit a chuckle. Dr. O'Leary smiles but doesn't laugh.

"You're in the superior range in terms of your verbal abilities."

So that's good, considering what I do for a living, I think. *At least I still have my words.*

Dr. O'Leary continues in a matter-of-fact way, her voice still weak from the illness she had last week, which I worry I might catch because I'm taking an immunosuppressant. "One of the tests that we looked at, that you had difficulty with was called working memory and that is holding information in your mind and manipulating it."

"Is that short-term memory?"

"That is kind of, yes, it is short-term memory, it overlaps a lot with it, there's kind of a formal definition for it. ... Digit-span forward is how many numbers can you hold in your mind. And you only had four. Actually, your digit-span backwards was better in that it was five."

My processing speed, Dr. O'Leary says, is "very high" but, by contrast, with multitasking, I score in the average range on the exams. On the matter of attention, she says, "We looked at sustained attention, which means for thirteen minutes can you stay focused?"

"Is that that test with the X? Oh, I was terrible at that!" This is a test where I sat in front of a laptop and was told to hit the space bar whenever the letter X appeared on the screen. Other letters, and sometimes numbers, appeared at a wide variety of intervals. Sometimes they appeared within a couple of seconds of another. Other times there were large gaps between appearances. After long gaps, I impulsively hit the space bar as soon as anything appeared, regardless of whether it is an X or not. I cursed aloud when I screwed up and impatiently hit the space bar. I know I don't do well, especially near the end.

"Yes, that's the X test," Dr. O'Leary says. "Your scores were in the average range. They weren't great, the twenty-seventh percentile ... I would say there is a little bit of an attentional vulnerability, not affecting how quickly you can do things but affecting your capacity to stay focused."

I am having some difficulties taking in new information, as well as with memory, she tells me, throwing in a token compliment about how my vocabulary, as measured by the Boston Naming Test, is strong.

Then Dr. O'Leary gets to that timed, name-all-the-words-that-start-with-the-letter-F test.

"Oh, that was awful," I grumble, embarrassed by the memory of how I froze for a couple of seconds as I attempted to grasp the question the young physician was asking.

"It wasn't awful," Dr. O'Leary counters. "It was average."

"It's funny because ... [the examiner] would say, 'name all the words that start with F,' and I'm thinking, 'ALL the words? There's no way, that's impossible, I don't think I CAN name ALL the words,' so I think I kind of I psyched myself out. But I'm not saying the results aren't accurate ..."

"But they may not be," Dr. O'Leary interrupts, "... it may have been that you got stuck on the instruction. ... There are some mild inefficiencies in terms of attention, otherwise, a very strong memory." She adds, "There's no impairment."

"Good!" I explode with enthusiasm, seeking something, anything, to indicate that all is not lost, that I won't, at least in the immediate future, slip away from myself as I have had enough of people and things slipping away from me lately, thank you very much. I want Dr. O'Leary to boost my confidence, to tell me good things. I crave them. Part of me knows this is an unrealistic expectation; her job is to explain the results, not to provide me with therapy. The other part of me does not care; it wants what it wants.

"You're clearly in the average range, it's just that it's not as good as you are smart and that may be sort of your longstanding pattern," Dr. O'Leary says, just before adding that I may struggle with multitasking and my working memory. The pre-MS Meredith boasted about being a multitasker extraordinaire. In college, I preferred to study in the middle of a bustling on-campus coffee shop. The ambient buzz of the activity seemed to enhance my concentration, whereas studying in a silent library made me fall asleep. I learned how to write news stories under tight deadlines in newsrooms where the chatter of other reporters, the sounds of the police scanners, and the ringing of the phones provided busy white noise.

As a freelance writer in my home office, I frequently had either cable TV news or talk radio playing in the background while I worked, as my kids loudly scampered around. I despise trying to work in silence. I need noise, the sound of life all around me when I am in the process of creating. But now that nerves in my brain have been damaged, likely irreparably, Dr. O'Leary is telling me my days of multitasking, of having a noisy bustle comfortably stimulating my thoughts, are over.

Not only should I knock off playing National Public Radio while I'm trying to correct dozens of news analyses for my journalism classes, I should take other measures to help me concentrate. When speaking with someone, Dr. O'Leary tells me I should avoid passive listening. I should interrupt people when they're speaking and ask questions like an over-caffeinated TV interviewer in order to increase the likelihood that I will remember the details of the conversation, she says. "Anything you do will slow them down, will make them repeat what they're saying, and will give you a second pass at the information," she says.

"The kids will love that," I reply. "'I've been told to interrupt you and ask you to repeat what you said.'" They already accuse me of acting like an investigative reporter digging for dirt whenever I ask them something as benign as, "How was English class today? What are you reading? Who did you eat lunch with today?" Being told to ramp up my inquiries will only yield serious eye-rolling, at least from Jonah and Casey.

Dr. O'Leary emits a courtesy laugh. I can't tell if she has a sense of humor or is simply humoring me. "One thing that people don't know is that when you repeat information … anything you want to learn, we all do better hearing something twice," she says.

We discuss what else I can do to compensate for my "mild" deficiencies: I should anticipate fatigue ("plan your schedule so that you can complete difficult tasks first"). I should avoid starting a new activity when I'm tired, I should get regular exercise, write down information as much as possible, and utilize apps on my iPhone for notetaking. Taking photos with the phone will also help jog my memory, she says. When I mention that Dr. Walker has raised the prospect of ADHD medications, she demurs, says she doesn't think I need it, at least not immediately.

"You seem very together," she comments.

Some vehicles have a warning written on the passenger side mirror that says: Objects are closer than they appear. If I were to have a warning imprinted on me, it might be this: Woman is not nearly as together as she may appear.

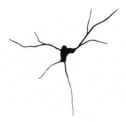

CHAPTER SEVENTEEN
Fatigue Factor

Fatigue: a case study. How does MS fatigue affect a forty-seven-year-old patient with relapsing remitting multiple sclerosis two years after her diagnosis? A study through anecdotes:

The high school cross country meet is not easily accessible. It's located atop what looks like a mountain top looming above the parking area at this central Massachusetts regional high school. There are paved, steeply inclined pathways that loop up the highland. Once you get to the end of that pathway, there's one more obstacle: two sets of very steep concrete stairs leading to the track on the flattened top of the earthen mound.

I walk very slowly. Ascending stairs, particularly several sets of stairs in a row, as well as scaling hills, are now things that turn my MS-addled thighs to Jell-O, rapidly weakening the limbs, and sending electrical signals buzzing through the legs like a colony of bees. Pre-MS Meredith didn't have this experience. Climbing stairs and walking up inclines never used to slay me like this. It was never fun, but it wasn't something I found thoroughly exhausting or challenging. It never made me feel like I was wading through mud. But this is not before. This is after.

Praying silently that no parents ask me what's wrong or why I'm walking in a way that suggests I'm recovering from an injury, I pace myself. I do not feel like blurting out, "I have

MS" to every person who looks at me quizzically. Nonetheless, I need to be able to make it to the top of these stairs. I want to see my two boys run in their cross country meet. I've already had to bail on events or on parts of events because stairs have proven to be an impediment. It is humiliating to have to do that, especially in front of the kids.

In the summer of 2016, I accompany Jonah and Abbey on college campus tours, usually led by students whose energy is as boundless as the wind. They rapidly walk-and-talk, like they are characters sprung to life from *The West Wing*. They have designated locations to hit and a limited timeframe in which to corral the group of parents and would-be students from place to place. They walk fast. They climb stairs even faster.

The first time this is a problem is when we are at Northeastern University in Boston. We go up and down several sets of stairs in a few buildings, and chase after the tour guide as he leads us across Huntington Avenue to show us a dorm. When I learn the group will be climbing yet more stairs in order to take a peek at a dorm room, I tell the kids I can't go with them. If I want to have enough oomph to make it to the end of the tour, I need a break. Feeling decades older than my forties, I collapse onto a bench as my legs tingle. I watch the tour group head up the stairs. My energy been depleted. I need rest. I felt like weeping, but I hold back the tears because I feel self-conscious enough having to drop out of the tour to sit on a bench and recover.

A similar thing occurs at UMass-Amherst. After a brisk walk across campus from the Visitors Center to the Tower Library in the full sun on a July morning, I feel nauseous when the chipper, bearded tour guide leads the group inside the library, down a flight of stairs and up a flight of stairs at a rapid clip. Trying to climb the dual sets of stairs at the tour guide's pace, even in the air-conditioned library, proves painful for me. I find lifting my legs harder and harder with each step. I drop to the back of the group. Eventually, I catch up with them when they pause in front of the Campus Center, in the blazing sunshine.

Can't we stand in some shade? I silently plead.

I notice flashing spots in the upper outside corners of my eyes as I quietly retch, my heat-sensitivity ramping up.

I'm going to faint, I think as my legs threaten to give out beneath me.

I hear the guide say he's taking the group across the street to some dorms. That's it for me. I bail, retreat into the air-conditioned Campus Center, sip a bottle of water, sit down, and feel like a loser, unable to keep up with my children, or the other parents.

Life is literally passing me by.

But at this cross country meet in the fall of 2016, I do not want to be that person, the one who's huffing and puffing, the one who looks woozy, the one who is unable to walk any further, the one who is missing out on parts of her children's lives. The weather is mild today, so I'm not in any danger of getting overheated and experiencing a temporary, temperature-related attack. For that I'm grateful. I strategically decide not to fight the multiple sclerosis. I will work with it, alongside it. (Fighting, I'm starting to realize, is a huge waste of my limited energy.) I will pace myself, do whatever is necessary to make it to that field and cheer on high school senior Jonah and high school sophomore Casey. I haven't been able to attend many of their sporting contests due to the twin obstacles of weather and MS fatigue. When factors are in my favor—the weather is good, the humidity is low, my energy level is decent—I need to show the kids that I can be there. I can still be their mother, their biggest fan. I haven't felt like I've been very good at that lately.

On this cloudy Saturday morning, with Scott watching high school senior Abbey at her cross country meet at another venue, I am here, determined to watch our boys. I may not be the fastest parent making my way up that mini-mountain. I may not look graceful, but I get up there. I cheer, obnoxiously loudly—much to Casey's mortification—and they hear me, nodding subtly in my direction to acknowledge me, hoping the nod shuts me up. Although I need to lie down and rest when I get home, for the moment I am standing next to that track, I am satisfied. My heart is full.

⁓

It is a work-in-progress, this learning how to be present with my family in our new circumstances. My therapist, who helps me work through my anxiety about my ambiguous future, gives me tools for this, as does Dr. Walker.

I learn coping techniques on how to deal with heat, like being okay with passing up events when it's expected to be hot and humid and I don't anticipate being able to get relief. I become the queen of the layered outfit, with sleeveless shirts or dresses as the base item of nearly any ensemble I wear, year-round, in New England. I drink cold drinks year-round as well, my favorite being a Dunkin' Donuts iced hazelnut coffee which yields raised eyebrows when I walk around with iced coffee on a 20-degree February day. When I'm teaching a university class in a room where I *can* control the thermostat—which actually happens during the spring 2017 semester—I drop the temperature down to 68 and overhear a student gripe to another, "Why is it always so damn *cold* in here?"

As much as it wounds my ego, I take naps—which I've taken to calling my "disco naps" if, for no other reason, than to annoy my sons who think me deeply nerdy—on days when I'm planning on going out in the evening. If I can help it, I try not to fill my hours with a series of consecutive, out-of-the-house events in order to be able to enjoy myself later in the day.

Of course, there are times when I lapse into old habits, cling to the vestiges of my former life and pretend, like a deluded idiot, that MS hasn't placed restrictions on my life. Take Christmas 2016 for example. Over the course of a couple of days after my MFA classes and the journalism class I teach are done for the semester, I plunge into a baking frenzy. I bake dozens of homemade cookies and desserts—peanut butter cookies topped with chocolate kisses, thumbprint cookies with jam centers, blinged-out sugar cookies, and a cranberry upside-down cake—not because I am going to be giving them out or having a lot of people over, but just because I haven't been doing a lot of baking and am trying to make up for lost time. During these same few days, I do a lot of shopping, wrap all the Christmas presents, and prepare homemade dinners each night. I also stay up later than I know I should.

And I pay the price for not pacing myself.

The night of Jonah's high school's holiday concert—where he plays drums with the jazz band and the chorus, as well as other percussion instruments with the wind ensemble—the impact of back-to-back days of unremitting activities unwittingly erects an impermeable wall through which I cannot pass. As I lean against an actual wall listening to members of the high school chorus, dressed in Dickensian holiday finery, sing ethereal Christmas tunes in the high school lobby, I realize I can go no further. I need to go home. Immediately. I honestly don't think I can stand up much longer as my body seems to be collapsing in on itself. My eyes droop and my vision is blurry. I have a conversation with a fellow music parent and, minutes later, have no idea what either of us said. Even carrying on a conversation with Scott as he drives me back to the house seems stunningly difficult, as does scaling the single flight of stairs from the first floor to the second, to get to my bedroom. For the next two days, I lie in bed while CNN anchors prattle on in the background about the latest unbelievable developments in U.S. politics. I slowly rebound, supposedly wiser, recognizing I stupidly pushed it too far.

That new-found knowledge about the repercussions of

doing too much is reinforced two months later in February 2017 when Scott and Abbey are in Florida to watch the Red Sox during spring training. I come home from the university after teaching on a Monday afternoon when my body hands me a receipt, demanding payment for me overscheduling the preceding weekend, for cramming too many things into those two days (yoga, shopping, cooking, writing, driving my sons around) without taking time to rest. I collapse onto the white sofa in our orange sunroom and don't move for several hours. My limbs are leaden. Facing the never-ending specter of an unmade dinner and lacking the physical will to talk the boys through making something, I hand Casey a twenty-dollar bill and say, "Get Jonah to take you someplace and buy yourselves dinner. Go wherever you want." Unlike with Christmas, I don't push any further, I just stay on that sofa, trying to remind myself that tomorrow it would most likely be better.

And it is.

Life with MS now means I must persuade myself to accept that I cannot attend the kids' coed Saturday night indoor soccer games, at which my parent friends bond over mugs of beer inside a glass-walled bar on the second floor overlooking the turf field while half-watching the teens play below. I bow out more times than I'm able to attend. I skip Casey's hockey games when they're scheduled for late in the evening and happen to be located a healthy drive away from the house. I pass up a couple of ladies' nights at a local brewpub and spur-of-the-moment meals if it's after eight and my energy level is in the danger zone. It's like that drive-at-your-own-risk dashboard light which turns when you're low on gas: best not to head into an area with heavy traffic and no gas stations. My energy level is something I can replenish with only one thing: sleep.

↩

I'm in the throes of last-minute editing for the book about the jazz band in mourning. My publisher has asked me to make some quick alterations which require me to scour the entire manuscript. I lock myself in my office over a weekend to make the changes, to triple-check the spelling on the front and back covers, and to greenlight the promotional material.

I'm wildly thrilled that *Mr. Clark's Big Band* is about to be published, that it will be in actual people's hands, specifically, in the hands of the classmates of Eric Green—the boy who passed away in seventh grade—a month before they graduate from high school in June 2017. That it will be in my son Jonah's hands, as the loss of his friend hit him hard and hit him deeply, creating a wound I could never help heal. It has felt like a sacred mission, getting this project done, doing literary justice to the year I observed that middle school band. Propelled by a missionary's zeal, I push through the hurdles, specifically, the cognitive and attention issues that Dr. O'Leary explained, which menace me just as I'm *thisclose* to completion.

Every time I take my MS medication, visit my neurologist, cannot focus, when my vision is filled with sparkly lights, and my thoughts are blurred by pounding head pain, when I am so tired that I cannot get out of bed, I think about my goal: finish the book and get it published. The book represents breaking through the yellow tape at the end of a marathon. I can see that tape now; it's in my sights. I am brusquely shunning other aspects of my life aside in order to get this done, getting shuteye even when I have a million things to do, hoping if I store my energy, I, ultimately, will cross that finish line.

My house, while relatively tidy, is not all that clean these days if you look beyond first impressions. I notice the dog hair on the carpet. I see dust darkening the white woodwork. The empty red window boxes that sit neglected beneath my front windows. There's chipped burgundy paint in the family room. The lavender paint in the hallway that's been there since we moved in in 2004 still needs to go. I avert my eyes to it all.

If I attend to these things, I can't finish the book, I remind myself.

I am having groceries delivered to the house more often than usual, however it seems I cannot keep enough food in the house as the three teenagers in residence scarf it down with startling speed. Casey, fifteen, is always griping about how we "have nothing" to eat after all the ready-to-eat items have disappeared. I pretend not to hear his complaints, although I do hear them, and they sting, and make me feel like a negligent mother. On at least two occasions, I order groceries when I am overtired and not thinking clearly. In those cases, I wind up with surprises inside the shopping bags, like the time there were two, thirty-two-ounce-bottles of white vinegar and two, thirty-two-ounce bottles of cranberry juice, a preposterously large amount of vinegar for a family that neither makes pickles nor uses vinegar for cleaning, and a ridiculously small amount of juice for a family of five. When Abbey and Scott extract the vinegar and cranberry juice bottles from the delivery bags, they exchange quizzical looks. After Abbey shows me the bottles, I guffaw loudly and for a bit longer than seemed entirely reasonable. "God, you really ARE tired," she says, as she shakes her head.

Health-conscious parents who have time and energy to prepare well-rounded meals for their growing children would be appalled at what I am passing off as dinner these days. A dinner comprised of appetizers (pigs in a blanket, spring rolls, pot stickers ... I know, all those preservatives ... *I know*), along with a side of sliced apples (hey, at least there's fresh fruit). Sometimes I pop frozen pizza in the oven and tell them when to take it out when it's done and serve themselves. On other nights, when my fuel gauge is getting close to that low-fuel warning, I make a quick breakfast-for-dinner like scrambled eggs, toast and sausage, or pancakes. We are having a disconcerting amount of pasta smothered with jarred marinara sauce. About two to three times a week I make something that I would be willing to serve to company, but on all the other nights, it's a makeshift combination of whatever we have in the house and how much steam I have in the tank to put the ingredients together.

Sadly, in these days leading up to the publication of *Mr. Clark's Big Band* and I'm also trying to complete a thesis to cap my MFA studies, Scott is not home in time to make dinner or misses dinner entirely because of work and/or because he's driving Casey to a later-evening hockey practice or game. I have donned blinders and am trying to focus on the goal. I need to block everything else out.

This means sacrificing holiday meals in the early months of 2017, taking shortcuts. Easter dinner, for example, is brunch at a local restaurant, instead of a buffet of homemade rack of lamb, a ham studded with cloves, asparagus with homemade Hollandaise sauce, roasted potatoes with rosemary, and home-made desserts like my mother used to serve. I long to bake the meat-laden Easter bread with chorizo, a Spanish sausage, that both my mother and her mother before her made, but I simply cannot do it this year and for that, I feel remorse. I don't want all the rituals with which I grew up to disappear simply because multiple sclerosis is in the picture.

Meanwhile, I'm unhealthily connected to my iPhone which, essentially, helps me run my post-MS life. It's like having an electronic brain that rapidly consumes energy and needs to be refueled, just like its owner. The phone reminds me to pick up Casey at the high school because I need to drive him to lacrosse practice in the neighboring town. It tells me there's a home track meet for Jonah tomorrow at four o'clock, that I need to call the vet at Healthy Paws to refill Max's pre-scription for heartworm pills, that I have to put together a gift basket to donate to my church's annual auction, that I have to get up *right now* because the yoga class I've recently started attending again is in less than an hour, that it's time to take my evening dose of medication, that the deadline to submit grades for the journalism class I teach is fast approaching. The phone alerts me several times daily that I need to attend to components of my life in a way in which I had never needed prompting.

I imagine my mother being dismayed by all of this. Dismayed that I haven't been putting up seasonal decorations on a regular basis, haven't been cooking that much, that my house needs a thorough cleaning, that my nails are bare, that my clothes aren't pressed, that my hair always seems to be in a messy ponytail. I imagine her tsk-ing and raising her well-groomed eyebrows as she surveys my life. Mom always threw a spotlight on things in my life—usually domestic and cosmetic—that she thought needed my attention, parceling out well-meaning maternal advice.

When I had a baby who didn't yet sleep through the night, plus a three-year-old twins, Mom came to spend the day with us while Scott was at work. She noticed that the fabric which covered the seats of the kitchen chairs I inherited from a great aunt, was stained. All the chair covers were in dire need of replacing.

"You know, recovering these chairs is really easy," Mom said, as she pulled a seat off its chair base and examined where the faded, 1970s-era olive-colored fabric was attached to the wood by staples.

I shrugged and turned my attention to Casey's diaper which I sniffed to determine if it needed changing. Sleep-deprived in those days, I was barely rallying myself to brush my hair and teeth each day. I honestly didn't care about the chairs, as sorry as they may have looked. I had many other things crowding my mind. Upholstering was not one of them. I was still potty-training one of the kids and had to figure out how to get them to nap, or play quietly, at least once a day so Casey could nap as well.

Nonplussed by my indifference, Mom pressed on. "I could help you do it. We could pick out fabric. It's really easy."

I should have known that resistance was futile.

"That's nice Mom, but I can't do it right now."

Yeah, I decided, *Casey needs to be changed.*

Weeks after her trial balloon, Mom took another day off from work to visit me and her grandkids again. (I was still on my break from teaching journalism in college since giving birth to Casey.) She coyly suggested the five of us go out to "get some air," to go someplace. I was up for that, if she agreed to strap the three-year-olds into their car seats, something that could be a struggle when they provided arched-back resistance. She readily agreed. However, fresh air was not on her itinerary. After plying me with a large coffee from the drive-through at Honey Dew Donuts, and buying the twins some doughnut holes, she persuaded me to drive to a fabric store in the neighboring town. With Abbey and Jonah sitting in their double-wide stroller and Casey safely buckled into in a baby carrier on my back, Mom seemed thoroughly delighted as we picked out a red and white plaid fabric that matched my Waverly kitchen curtains. Hours later, the stained, faded, and worn original olive covers on the hand-me-down chairs were history.

Mom smiled triumphantly. "See, that wasn't so hard. They look great!"

I grinned back, wanting to please her but doing a poor job of feigning my enthusiasm. She was right, they did look great. The new covers were a vast improvement over the old ones. But, just as I feared, it wasn't long before several of the new seat covers became soiled, hapless victims of dollops of grape jelly squeezed out of PB&J sandwiches by chubby pre-schooler hands, smeared with melted chocolate ice cream, and dotted with marinara sauce that slid down a strand of overcooked spaghetti as it dangled from Jonah's mouth. I didn't have the heart to tell Mom. With three kids under the age of four, stains were to be expected. We would have been better off waiting to re-recover the chairs, but I couldn't tell her that. She wanted things to look good for her family. I made efforts to hide the stains whenever she visited.

Years later, after I moved to my current home and once my children reached middle school, Mom noticed that the textured gray seat covers on my three kitchen stools had a few darkened spots. The covers were fully intact. The stools were fairly new, but the locations where olive oil and other mystery substances had been resistant to my vigorous scrubbing were noticeable.

"Have you ever thought about recovering these stools?" Mom asked.

Internally, I rolled my eyes. Externally, I changed the subject.

We ... rather, *she* never got around to cajoling me into recovering the stools—they remain their glorious, stained selves to this day—but I still hear her voice, directing my attention to them as I clean up after the kids. The house will never be pristine, not until the kids move out. And I'm totally okay with that.

I still hear Mom's voice when I notice that the windowsills in my bedroom need painting, that furniture needs dusting, that the yard would certainly look better with some perennials and a bit (a lot) of weeding out front. Mom was a diligent, dedicated gardener. Me, I hate gardening. There were many visits when she offered me advice on how to improve my flower beds at the old house, how to keep the flowers in the window boxes in my new house from dying. Problem was, these things were not priorities to me.

Mom's voice morphs inside my head, chastises me for my slackery which, with multiple sclerosis, seems much more pronounced than ever before. I wonder what she would say if she had lived to see this new version of me, this MS-afflicted person who cannot keep up with the standards of cleanliness set by her, by my grandmother Olivia, and my great-grandmother Maria, who was infamous for moving her refrigerator once a week and cleaning behind it.

I have a vivid memory of Gram babysitting Sean and me for the weekend while my parents went to Newport. "Wouldn't it be fun to wash and wax the kitchen floor to surprise your mother?" she asked me, a grade schooler to whom washing and waxing a kitchen floor did not seem fun as I jealously eyed Sean who escaped such drudgery by the mere fact that he wasn't a girl and wasn't expected to clean anything.

Couple this with the reputations my great grandmother, Gram, and Mom had for entertaining and cooking, and I knew I would never live up to their standards. Great Grandma made multiple main dishes for holiday meals and watched over you as you ate, looking for signs you had anything other than a positive reaction to her food. Gram would likewise prepare mountains of food for family meals and would push the food like a drug dealer, even if you told her if you ate any more you'd vomit.

When I start to castigate myself for not living up to the measures set by my maternal ancestors, I pause, and consciously try to quell the critical voices before they reduce me to an insecure twentysomething who's just learning how to be an adult and keep house. I try to distinguish, inside my head, how or whether the condition of my neat-but-not-exactly-clean house is similar or dissimilar from my father's house. It's all so confusing.

This isn't the 1940s, 1960s, the 1980s, I tell myself. My priorities are not the same. And that is okay. I'm doing the best I can. Time is my most valuable commodity right now.

Thus, I'm furiously plugging away at the eleventh-hour editing to what I thought was an already-finished manuscript. I spend hours to spread advance word about *Mr. Clark's Big Band*. I prep myself for interviews (for which I need to be clear-headed and well rested).

Reupholstering the kitchen stools will have to wait.

CHAPTER EIGHTEEN

Bickell Strong

The launch party I'm planning just before *Mr. Clark's Big Band's* May 2 publication date is roiling my innards. Everything about it intimidates me. The size and scope of it. Its public nature, as it's going to be held in the middle school where the book takes place. Over a hundred people respond to their Evites and say they plan to attend. Many of the students I observed during the 2012-2013 school year, the ones who were friends and bandmates of Eric Green, are on the invitation list, as are current middle school members of the Big Band, my Southborough friends, my college buddies, my father, my uncle, my brother and his family.

I am slated to explain how the book came into being, what went into the researching and writing of it (sans the explanations about project delays due to my mother's death, my father's difficulties, and my illness). Then I'll read excerpts. Jamie Clark is also expected to speak, and the explosive sounds of jazz are to follow when the students, current and former, perform. Afterward, I'll be called upon to sign copies of the book, finished copies of which are supposed to arrive at my house in time, according to my publisher. But two weeks before the book launch party, they haven't yet been delivered. I have yet to see a final copy of the book.

Did the last-minute edits I made make it to my publisher? Will the books get here in time?

When I distribute the electronic invitations, I write that there will be "light refreshments" to disabuse anyone of the notion that they will be getting lunch at this 1 p.m. soiree.

The food! There will be a lot of teenagers there. How much should we get? What should we get? I start asking. *Should I get flowers for tables? And what about tablecloths?*

I break into flop sweat. As they witness my rising panic, Scott and my friend Deb, a fellow band parent, benevolently and gently inform me that they will take over the event planning or, at least, the food and decorations portion.

"I just want you to show up and speak," Scott tells me one night after a typical so-so dinner I hastily whip together after I drive Casey to and from his lacrosse practice, and after having taught my journalism class in Boston earlier in the day. We are sitting at the kitchen table which, I notice, still has crumbs on it. The kids are supposed to clean up after supper. They do. Kind of. Except for these crumbs.

Just ignore it, I say silently.

I rub my eyes, forgetting that I haven't yet removed my makeup. Remnants of mascara darken the pads of my fingers. Make-up can no longer camouflage my exhaustion. All the so-called magical eye makeup remedies I ordered online are powerless against this kind of lethargy. The whole world can see my fatigue now. Even though people may not know that I have multiple sclerosis—not many people know this fact yet—it's painfully clear that I'm run down.

After I meet with Jamie to discuss the details of the book launch party, he texts me soon afterward. "Quick question ... Everything ok?" he writes, saying his "radar" is telling him all is not well with his writer friend. His radar is right.

Scott sees it too and is trying to "fix it" or at least make sure the launch party succeeds. "I'm going to keep you in the loop, ask you to check off on stuff, but I don't want you to worry about the food or decorations," he says. "Deb and I have you covered."

I tear up and wrap him in a fraught embrace. Two-year-old Tedy barks his incessant, high-pitched bark, demanding to be included in the hug.

I am so very grateful that Scott and Deb have taken charge. Even considering the reduction in my energy post-MS, I'm in particularly rough shape.

I am having trouble sleeping again. I lie in bed at night and run through the order of events for the book launch. While curled on my side and facing the windows, wishing I could go to sleep, I start writing my speech, trying out lines. This leads to me to start imagining all the things that could go wrong, which brings me to lifelike scenes of me being publicly felled by MS symptoms, like fainting, being stricken by vision issues, dizziness, and vomiting at this big moment of celebration, imagining everyone witnessing my disease-induced weaknesses in full, like being wheeled out on a stretcher in my black cotton nightgown and loaded into an ambulance in full view of my neighbors. That naked vulnerability, that image, makes frequents appearances in my dreams.

I need to be rested, I tell myself while I lie there and shake off the worries. It's no use. I keep worrying. *Will the room be too hot? Will I have a heat reaction? Maybe Jamie can help with that?*

While I can plan for a lot of aspects of this book party, one thing I cannot guarantee is what my body may do. I start thinking of that 1980 "This is your brain on drugs" public service ad but with a twist: "Okay, last time ... This is your body. This is MS." I picture me, on my bathroom floor, crippled by vomiting, dizziness, and head pain, fainting, being hospitalized. "Any questions?"

When I can no longer stay in bed and soak in my own anxiety, I retreat to the family room downstairs and turn something stupid on the TV to distract me, anything to get me off this never-ending carousel of concerns.

This is not good, this not getting sleep. It is analogous to knocking over the first of a line of dominos. If I don't sleep, I will get overly fatigued. If I am overly fatigued, I will get headaches, sometimes debilitating ones, along with eye pain that render me unable to read. The combination of these factors will hinder my ability to concentrate which will stress me out further, which could lead to me not being able to carry on with the work I need to do in the limited time in which I have to do it.

Someone please stop my brain from thinking all these anxious thoughts! It's like If You Give a Mouse a Cookie, *but on steroids.*

After all these years, Scott can read me well. His telling me that he will take care of the food and decorations for this shindig is an incredibly kind gift. I take it and grab it like a greedy child on Christmas morning and keep my roiling mental morass to myself.

~

I'm in one of those post-yoga bliss moments.

While I grouchily drag myself out of bed at seven forty-five on Saturday mornings and hastily don yoga-appropriate clothes in order to make it to my eight-thirty yoga class in time, it's almost always worth it. I feel lighter in the hours just after the practice concludes, full of possibilities. If my instructor is in a playful mood and pushes the class to be overzealous with our yoga positions—going deeply in the poses, holding them a tad too long—I typically start feeling the painful after-effects by late afternoon. But in the immediate aftermath, I am a walking rainbow, which is the opposite of my current mental state.

It is sunny and relatively warm on this April Saturday morning, but the temperature suits me fine. I sit down at the kitchen table with a pile of newspapers from the week that I haven't had the chance to read yet. Fresh hazelnut coffee sits in my "Trust me, I'm a reporter" mug. It does not taste burnt, indicating some of my taste irregularities may have waned.

My morning is a Hallmark ad. While perusing an edition of the *New York Times* from a few days ago, I see a story about a thirty-one-year-old hockey player who made a triumphant return to the NHL after having been diagnosed with multiple sclerosis.

The Carolina Hurricanes' Bryan Bickell, I learn, had been experiencing an array of peculiar physical difficulties for a long period of time. Those difficulties came crashing down on him in late October 2016 when he lost "function in his right arm and leg during a morning skate," Bickell told the *Times*. The man who'd been a member of three Stanley Cup-winning teams, the man with a wife, baby, and preschooler at home, was told he had the disease without a cure. As Bickell explained to ESPN, "It was just all of a sudden. It was my right side of my body. My right arm, my right leg were kind of disconnected." He also experienced problems with balance and with his vision.

Intrigued by this story that depicted Bickell in a heroic, man-overcomes-adversity tale, I start to research more about him: his symptoms began to fade once he began receiving an MS drug administered via IV every four weeks and he returned to the Hurricanes' minor league team for practices in late January. "With the treatments I'm getting, every month it's getting on the ice and working hard to get my game somewhere close to getting back in the lineup," Bickell told *The News & Observer* before he returned to the NHL in early April. "The progress is going the right way and that's what we've been looking forward to the past couple of months."

On April 4, 2017, Bickell, a six-foot-four, youthful-looking man with a neat, reddish-brown full beard, and short, well-coifed hair, became the third NHL player with multiple sclerosis to take to the ice. In the *Times* article headlined "After an M.S. Diagnosis, an Emotional Return to the N.H.L. Ice," I learn about the two other NHL players who'd had multiple sclerosis, both goaltenders who didn't have to constantly skate up and down the ice, but had to remain standing, with no break, for long stretches of time. Josh Harding played "parts of two seasons" with the Minnesota Wild and "retired after collapsing during a minor league game," the *Times* said. The other player, Jordan Sigalet, "spent three seasons in the minors, made one, 43-second appearance for the Boston Bruins in January 2006, then played briefly in Europe before retiring in 2009," the paper reported.

As I read about Bickell's comeback, a fresh thread of hope runs through me. Maybe it's the byproduct of my yoga class, maybe it's the caffeine in my second cup of coffee, but the Bickell tale resonates strongly. I read the article again and call Scott over. "Look at this," I say, "this thirty-one-year-old hockey player was just diagnosed with MS and he's already back to playing."

I try to imagine what that's like. Skating up and down the ice. Sweating profusely under the many layers of pads and protective gear. Hair slick with perspiration.

How does he keep himself cool enough? I wonder. *How does he sustain his energy? Maybe it's the medication. ... I mean, if he can fully participate in an NHL game ...*

The discussion about Bickell piques Casey's interest. He has been playing hockey since grade school. He is hanging around in the family room while Scott and I are pouring over the articles in the adjacent kitchen. "That's great Mom," he says genuinely. "Very cool."

I feel compelled to seek out Jonah and Abbey, each of whom is in their own bedroom doing homework. I tell them about Bickell too. It suddenly seems important to me, a vital a piece of information I feel they need to have, although I cannot say why, exactly, other than it creates new possibilities for my future. Bickell's story reaches deep into my chest and gently cups my heart. If he can return to hockey, then maybe my multiple sclerosis won't eventually push me into a downward spiral where my ability to function, to do the work that I love, will erode.

The next day, a Sunday, while checking Twitter, I enter "Bickell" into the search engine and see the hashtag #Bickell-Brave in the search results. I discover that, while Bickell was speaking at a charity walk to raise money for MS research, Hurricanes teammates and staffers surprised him by joining the walk while wearing white "#BickellBrave" T-shirts with Bickell's number twenty-nine on the back. Videos showed him teary-eyed as he embraced the members of the Hurricane family. My heart feels full for this man I had never heard of before yesterday, this man who is a proxy for me, for my future.

"Hey, guys," I shout from the same spot at the kitchen table where I first read about Bickell's story, "look at this." For a moment, I'm unable to speak. My throat is tightening, salty tears flood my eyes and threaten to leak down my face. "That hockey player with MS ..." I manage to get out, "his teammates walked the MS Walk with him."

Like with everything related to multiple sclerosis since I involuntarily joined the ranks of the millions of people across the globe with the disease, the Bickell news seems intensely personal. This explains why, when Bickell announces he's going to retire from hockey, a week after donning his Hurricanes jersey after a four-month-long absence, the news hits me hard, prompting me to experience an odd sense of despair. I scour the internet looking for a reason *why*, after such a profoundly moving comeback, Bickell can't do it anymore. I need to know. I find an article on NHL.com which says, "The final decision to hang up the skates at the conclusion of the season was made in the last week after discussions with his wife and his parents. 'Hockey is not everything. I've got a life after hockey. To live a healthy life for the rest of my life is important for me and my family,' he said. 'We made the decision to [retire], and I won't take any regrets. I've had a pretty good career and made the best of it.'" He says he knew his body would never feel the same since being stricken with MS. Later in the article, Bickell tells the reporter, "It's been really emotional. I had some times breaking down, but that's part of who I am and just the passion behind this,' he said."

What happened exactly? I cannot find specific answers in the news articles. All I know is that, alongside the heartfelt words spoken about Bickell, the standing ovation the crowds gave him, the supportive hashtag on social media, multiple sclerosis took Bickell off the ice. The moment of hopeful optimism I experienced when I read that Bickell had returned, post-diagnosis, is extinguished like the fleeting light of a birthday candle, a silent wish made over the shadowy light that's not granted.

As the culmination of my book project gets closer, specifically the launch party, the more apprehensive I get that multiple sclerosis will ruin it for me, take me off my playing field. As much progress as I have made in trying to accept my post-MS limitations and alterations to my lifestyle, the road to making peace with this disease is winding.

‿

When I can sleep, I keep having these dreams. In them, a bunch of people unexpectedly drop by my house (only it's not my real house, it's a different house, but I own it). I scramble to whip up something for the faceless visitors to eat and drink. However, every time I go to serve the guests, I drop everything. The glasses slip out of my hands and red wine flows out from its initial splatter point and covers significant portions of the kitchen floor. The glass bowls of nuts or crackers or grapes (the contents vary by dream) also fall to the ground and shatter, sending the contents tumbling through the pools of wine.

Or I dream that I'm driving to the university but get irrevocably lost on the way, forget how to get there. I am marooned on the side of the road, alone, and do not know what to do.

GPS never figures into these dreams. An alternative version of the "lost" dream has me not only getting disoriented, but also learning that I have completely forgotten to attend some math classes I am supposed to take in order to get my MFA degree, classes in which I enrolled but simply never attended. On what's supposed to be graduation day, I learn I have failed. (In real life, graduation for me is in May.)

Forgetfulness. Clumsiness. An incapacity to do things right. Failing. In the light of day, I can process these doubts, apply rational thinking, and put them into their proper place. But every night when my head hits the pillow, my anxious brain doesn't care about rational thinking.

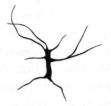

CHAPTER NINETEEN
Launch

Scott pulls together a posse, a group of our parent-friends, plus band director Jamie, and two administrators at the Trottier Middle School. Everybody, except for the two administrators, knows about my multiple sclerosis. They know about the fatigue thing. The overheating thing. The headaches ... all that fun MS stuff. That is why they are shifting into high gear, holding organizational meetings and exchanging group texts in order to plan the granular details of the book launch party. They know what went down in my life during the time I was researching, writing, editing, selling, and preparing the final version of the manuscript for publication. Many were witnesses to it. My friends Sharon, Deb, Gretchen, and Jamie attended my mom's wake, and helped organize meals for my family for over a week in the spring of 2014 after she died. Sharon was there with me in the hospital after the massive MS attack in July 2014, just before that ill-fated lumbar puncture, while Gretchen was busy saving Casey's thirteenth birthday. Deb and Jamie visited me while I was home recuperating after my hospitalization.

Now Scott calls upon these four, as well as other friends in town like Lise, with whom we went on vacation on Martha's Vineyard and whose father had MS, to help with this gathering for nearly 200 people. The total number of attendees seems to increase by the day. The posse is dividing the work amongst the volunteers, which even includes Eric Green's mother Suzy.

They refuse to burden me with any of it. It feels so strange, letting people take over the work. I may hate the sense of passivity I'm experiencing, prompting flashbacks of my mom rushing around before events doing everything herself. It may make me feel like a slacker, but it is imperative that I relinquish this work and focus. I am learning to take, "Yes" for an answer.

The book launch party and publication date are only a few days away and I can't shake this sense of foreboding that's warning me that multiple sclerosis will pull a nasty trick on me. Although Jamie has said he'll make sure the middle school cafeteria, where the party will be held, will be cool enough, temperature-wise, for me, I am haunted by visions of fainting at the podium, of my speech become slurred, of my concentration waning, knees buckling, vision obstructed by pre-migraine spots appearing in the periphery of my vision. Days before the event, those shiny, sparkling spots burst into my eyes after dinner one night. I can't read, look at my phone, or even watch TV for several hours.

What if that happens at or just before the party?

I've always experienced some degree of stage fright when faced with speaking in front of large groups, but I tend to quickly overcome it as soon as I dive into my remarks, which have usually been well rehearsed. Teaching in front of large college classes has, to some degree, prepared me for public speaking, but I haven't spoken in front of over one hundred people in my post-MS life. Worries that, during what should be a moment of celebration, multiple sclerosis will take me out the way it drove Brian Bickell out of the NHL, menace me.

⌒

I am returning from picking Casey up from school and am about to pull into my driveway when I notice a UPS truck has preceded me. It's a delivery guy with several boxes containing one hundred and fifty copies of *Mr. Clark's Big Band*. I open the garage door and direct the man inside, surprised to feel a rush of pride inside my chest.

"Big delivery," the guy says.

"There are copies of my new book in there," I say, taken aback by the delight in my voice. Everybody's been asking me if I'm *excited* about the book coming out, *excited* about the book launch party.

What I am, I want to tell them, *is nauseous and apprehensive.*

On occasion, I confess the truth to the person asking me the excitement question, but most of the time, I just smile and try to change the subject. But here in my driveway, as I watch this stranger unload the boxes containing the physical manifestation of a goal, years in the making, and place them inside my garage, *excitement* is exactly what I'm feeling. It's something I haven't experienced in so long that it feels unnatural.

Once the boxes are lined up, the man smiles and says, "That's really great." He even sounds like he means it as he adds, "Good luck to you."

⤴

The moment my eyes open on the morning of Sunday, April 30 and I remember that today is the day, I feel my stomach muscles clench. I lie still for a minute and assess. I have not contracted a stomach bug or any of the other viral and bacterial illnesses going around that might keep me from attending my own book launch party. I'm not feeling migraine or eye pain, or leg/ankle spasms. After I take silent inventory of how my body is feeling—other than the nervous stomach— I am surprised to find myself well.

Still, I am wary. There are several hours to go before I'm supposed to read my speech and excerpts from *Mr. Clark's Big Band* for the first time. So many things can go wrong between now and then.

Over the previous two days, I tried to sweeten my odds of things going my way. I kept a low profile, didn't go out much. I took a pass on a gathering of friends the night before the book party so I could rest up. And as much as the pre-MS Meredith would have insisted on being a part of the event planning, would have demanded that I participate in the making of the centerpieces, the setting up/preparing/ordering of the food, the arrangement of the balloons and the table linens, the post-MS Meredith is keenly aware that that's a stupid idea. In fact, it takes all the energy I have, after several days of keeping activity to a minimum, just to keep my nervousness contained, to write and review my speech and readings, to simply shower and get myself ready.

I walk into the middle school cafeteria about an hour before the event is to begin and discover that my posse—plus my kids and some of their friends—have it well covered. Green, white, and yellow balloons are tethered by white ribbons all around the room. There are round tables in the middle of the space covered by cream-colored tablecloths with a gold overlay and are dotted with shiny plastic musical note confetti. Glass vases filled with rolled up sheet music on cream-colored paper—the cover pages of three pieces the Big Band played during the year I shadowed them, pieces related to Eric Green—sit in the center of those tables as fresh sunflowers rise from within the sheet music. Wrapped around the middle of the vases: a thick burlap ribbon affixed with a heavy-stock, black tag bearing, handwritten in gold Sharpie, "When words fail, music speaks." The book table is covered with a green tablecloth, features more musical confetti and a vase with sheet music-wrapped sunflowers. Several long tables are lined up together along the other side of the room, tables that would soon groan with the weight of brownies, green and white cookies in the shape of musical notes, a giant fruit bouquet, and ample platters of cheese and crackers. In the corners of the room, balloon-festooned stands bear oversized, glossy images of the cover of *Mr. Clark's Big Band* mounted on card-board. One of the large poster boards has enlarged photos of Jamie conducting the Big Band while another has a collage of photos of the band students from the year I followed them. In the very front of the room, there are rows of stools, chairs, beat-up black music stands, a drum set, a large xylophone, and an upright piano ready for the current and alumni members of the Big Band to perform.

My husband, my kids and my friends did this, I think. *Wow, they did all of this.*

As people begin to fill the room, I wait for my stomach to ache, for me to be paralyzed by fear because I fervently don't want to let down Jamie, the band kids, fellow band parents, or Suzy Green, who picked out the flowers for the centerpieces. But a strange thing occurs. Instead of feeling as though I am being swallowed up by nerves and obsessing about the many way in which my body might fail me, I feel buoyed, light, a hot air balloon aloft looking down at the picturesque scenery.

I'm pleasantly shocked when I notice that Dad has arrived, along with his brother and his brother's wife. My brother Sean and one of my nephews are here, as are my college friends Gayle, Garron, Tim, and Kerry. My Southborough friends, especially those who magically transformed the atmosphere of the cafeteria with their deft creative touches, are beaming. In addition to the current middle school Big Band members, many alums, including those about whom I wrote, are in the room, all waiting to hear me read from excerpts of my book, the book about a very important slice of their lives.

The previous day, the only thing I did other than rest was attend Casey's JV lacrosse game at the high school. While I was sitting in the bleachers, I was speaking with my friend Amy, who has a daughter in the current Big Band as well as two older sons who previously participated in Jamie's band program. I told her I was apprehensive about the party, concerned I'd flub my speech.

"But these are your people," she said. "We've got your back."

My people.

My people.

My people AND my book. They are both here. And I am still standing.

‧৹

The school principal, Keith Lavoie, steps to the maple-colored podium and relates the tragic origins of this book, the loss of seventh grader Eric, the crushing grief experienced by Eric's classmates and teachers, how Jamie provided the students with compassion and tender guidance during a challenging period, and then how I entered the picture to tell their story.

"When [Eric] passed our community was tested and our resolve was measured," Keith says. "... In moments of tragedy, everyone wants to say or do something but they aren't quite sure what to say or what to do. I'm sure we can all relate to that in one way or another. But then when we have a moment, we take pause, we figure things out, amazing things can happen."

We figure things out.

As Keith calls me up to the microphone on the right side of the room, my edginess completely dissolves. In front of me is a community of friends and family. Behind me, the promise of young musicians and their beloved band director Jamie, the guy who I was interviewing when I experienced my very first MS symptoms in the summer of 2012. Surrounded, on all sides, by love, by people who had faith in this book, in me.

I do not fumble my speech—although Jamie, attempting to cool off the room as it grew stuffy, makes so much noise as he opens the doors behind the band and distributes chairs to the students who are standing that I pause, mid-sentence, and wait for him to finish arranging the furniture. Everyone laughs, as do I. It's such a Jamie Clark thing to do, to busy himself fixing things in the middle of an event. When Jamie finishes moving the furniture, I continue. I do not slur my words. I do not faint. My knees do not buckle. No one has to pick me up off of the floor because I am flying. I do not need to rely on the written speech; I already know it in my heart.

The middle school jazz musicians nail their four pieces before Jamie invites the Big Band alums to sit in, including Jonah on the drums, for the last piece, "Groovin' Hard." It is energetic, jubilant, joyful. After an encore where they play the last few, bombastic measures of "Groovin' Hard" again, the crowd heartily applauds their children, their band director, their music program, their community.

I am radiating uncharacteristic elation from my spot on the side of the room when I feel Jamie grabbing my right hand firmly in his left as he pulls me in front of the band. He sweeps his arms like a game show host toward me, encouraging the crowd to applaud. Momentarily horrified and stunned, I am a bashful schoolgirl standing there, uncertain about what I should do with my hands. Members of the crowd rise to their feet. A standing ovation. I've never had one of those before. Jamie, in his bright cornflower blue shirt which contrasts with my black dress, extends his arms and moves in for a bearhug. I hug him back and allow the warmth of everything to sink in, down to my bones. In this moment, I am not afraid of the warmth. It is sustaining me.

I'm going to be okay.

Acknowledgments

Surviving and thriving in the wake of the diagnosis of a chronic, incurable illness is not a solo endeavor. Neither is writing a book about the experience.

Throughout the process of writing *Uncomfortably Numb*, an early draft of which was my thesis for my Master of Fine Arts in creative nonfiction from Bay Path University, I received incredibly positive feedback from my thesis adviser, Adam Braver, and from my Bay Path classmates. All of them—particularly Jodie, Heidi, and Anne—asked just the right questions, offered sage advice, and helped me deepen and enrich my writing.

I am grateful to the people who provided me with information and clarification about MS, including my neurologist (whom I told I would not name in this book), and to Lori Espino, the chairwoman of the New England chapter of the National Multiple Sclerosis Society.

My husband Scott, whose life is very exposed on the pages of this work, told me to write whatever I felt I needed to, whatever my personal truth was. For a guy who doesn't like to share a lot of personal details about his life with others, this was a gift for which I am grateful.

My children—Abbey, Jonah, and Casey—helped fill in gaps in my memory and provided me with key details which helped me recreate family experiences affected by multiple sclerosis. They also helped boost my confidence when it waned. You three are blessings.

I also extend my appreciation to my brother Sean, who encouraged me to tell my story and not worry about anything else, and to my friend Gayle who also provided me with information and clarification about events described here.

Author's Note

While this is a work of nonfiction, it is a collection of my experiences as I remember them. It may not reflect everyone's truth. When writing scenes in this book, I often consulted with others who were also there to confirm my recollections and to add salient details. I also used contemporaneous notes, text messages, datebooks, and medical reports to help provide me with specifics.

In her memoir, *Pigs Can't Swim*, author Helen Peppe said: "I did my best to recreate dialogue out of the mush of thousands of conversations, my own and others, that were, again, mostly the same. I cannot guarantee that any scene or any conversation is a replica." What she said.

I changed the names of all the medical professionals I visited and do not identify the hospitals and medical facilities at which I received treatment. This is by design. *Uncomfortably Numb* is intended to provide a portrait of what it's like, from a patient's perspective, to be plunged into a confusing and extended diagnostic process, and then to cope with the aftermath of being told you have an incurable disease which may or may not strip you of your ability to walk, see, and think clearly.

As I researched multiple sclerosis, I referenced many sources which are directly cited in the book. I also heavily consulted the National Multiple Sclerosis Society's website, the National Institutes of Health website, the Mayo Clinic website, WebMD, Healthline, the Everyday Health website, the Multiple Sclerosis Association of America website, MultipleSclerosis.net, the Multiple Sclerosis News Today website, and *Multiple Sclerosis: New Hope and Practical Advice for People with MS and Their Families* by Louis J. Rosner and Shelley Ross.